D0402095

The Pursuit of Life

English version of the Chinese book entitled,
"Total Health of Body, Mind and Spirit,"
Torch of Wisdom, Taipei, 1992.

Chiu-Nan Lai, Ph.D.

Lapis Lazuli Light

The Pursuit of Life

Copyright © 1993 Chiu-Nan Lai, Ph.D.

All rights reserved. No part of this book may be reproduced by any means without prior written permission from the publisher.

Lapis Lazuli Light
P.O. Box 1795
Soquel, CA 95073
U.S.A.

Typography by BookPrep
Cover Design by Josh Gitomer
Silk embroidery of cranes and pine is from Xiantan, Hunan;
    both are symbols of longevity.
Printed in U.S.A.

ISBN: 0-9638477-0-8
Library of Congress Catalogue Card Number: 93-80034

Acknowledgments

This book chronicles twenty years of research and studying of healing around the world. Many people contributed to my education, from my initial introduction to Dr. Norman Walker's book on "Raw Vegetable Juices" through a college friend to studying with H.H. The Dalai Lama in 1987. I wish to express my heartfelt gratitude to all of them, especially Liane Crawford who facilitated my growth through sound and color; Goenkaje whose mind training technique in Vipassana Meditation changed my life; Lama Zopa Rinpoche, a healer of all levels; and of course H.H. The Dalai Lama who first "called" me "home" to Dharamsala, India where I studied for three years from 1987 to 1990. His presence was transformative.

I thank my parents, whose unconditional love provided the self-confidence that I needed to explore beyond limitations.

The original Chinese version of the book, entitled "Total Health of Body, Mind, and Spirit" was first published in April of 1992 by Torch of Wisdom (10, Lane 270, Chien Kuo S. Road Sec. 1, Taipei, Taiwan 10630, R.O.C.). It sold out seven printings in little over one year. Many of my English-speaking friends requested that I translate the book into English. My decision to do it came only after Dr. Arthur Hubbard, my closest friend and teacher of twenty years, offered to edit the English version. Thank you, Arthur, for all your love and support which prompted the publication of this English version.

This book is dedicated to the healing of our planet.

Table of Contents

Part I

Open-Heartedness

Chapter 1
Open-heartedness, the wellspring of health and good fortune

In Chinese, "open-heartedness" literally means joy and happiness. The play on these two words is difficult to preserve in translation.

Open-heartedness is the wellspring of health and good fortune. It is also the basic solution to problems of the individual, family, society and the world. This is the essential wisdom of the past and present. One sees many illustrations of this in Chinese medical knowledge and in the Chinese language itself.

In Chinese medicine there is an understanding of the negative influence on health of the seven emotions and six desires. Chinese medicine includes descriptions of how certain emotions affect certain organ systems. For example, anger hurts the liver, grief hurts the lungs, overjoyousness hurts the heart, fear hurts the kidneys, and worrying and obsessive thinking hurt the spleen. If one is in equanimity, then the Chi (life force) is calm; if the mind is relaxed then the body is well. Let us look more closely at the words "open-heartedness": If the heart is open then one is joyous and happy. When husband and wife meet each other their hearts are open and naturally they are happy. When we meet with our enemies, with strangers or encounter

3

unhappy situations the heart closes and we become unhappy. Also, when we are parted from our dear ones, the heart is closed and we become unhappy. Open-heartedness (happiness) and the heart being open are linked. If one wishes to have health and happiness, it is important to understand this link.

In 1981, under the U.S.-China scholarly exchange program, I made my first visit to Beijing to collaborate with the Chinese Cancer Institute. The research project was to investigate the causes for high rates of esophagus cancer in Linxian, in the Henan province of northeastern China. The incidence of esophagus cancer in that region is the highest of any region in China, and this is attributed to enviromental factors and dietary habits. Residents of Linxian are fond of pickled vegetables and moldy breads. The soil of Linxian is deficient in the mineral molybdenum, and this reduces the vitamin C content of the fruits and vegetables which grow there. All of these factors contribute to the development of the disease. Of course, not everyone in Linxian develops esophagus cancer. The people of Linxian have often had the experience that following a family conflict and subsequent feelings of anger, an individual would develop difficulty in swallowing. Upon medical check-up, cancer of the esophagus was diagnosed. This example illustrates that although enviromental and dietary factors contribute to cancer, the trigger was the loss of open-heartedness (loss of happiness).

Various medical studies have shown that emotions and illnesses are linked. Following the loss of a spouse, a person's immune response is often lowered for several months. People showing type A behavior, involving frequent emotional outburts, are more prone to heart attacks. Those with type B personalities, in which emotions are repressed are more prone to cancer. In western medicine, a new field is emerging involving the study of the link between the mind, immune system and nervous system, called Psycho-neuroimmunology.

In the following, I will report the experiences of two doctors which illustrate the relationship between open-heartedness and health and disease. Dr. R.G. Hamer is a specialist in Cancer in Cologne, Germany. In 1979, soon after their son was murdered in Italy, both he and his wife developed cancer. After this experience, Dr. Hamer changed his views in regard to the development of cancer. The development stage of cancer can be as short as a few months. Also emotional conflicts and shock are significant factors in the onset of cancer. After his new understanding of cancer, through working on the psychological level, he himself recovered from his cancer. He started to observe among his patients that before the onset of the illnesses, they had experienced a shock or an inner conflict about which they could not talk or there was no one to whom to talk. After talking out and resolving the initial conflict, the illness was reversed. Furthermore, by CT scanning, Dr. Hamer detected lesions in the brain, the locations of which depended on the nature of the conflict. A cancer was discovered later in a corresponding part of the body. He collected a total of 10,000 cases. His published work is available in German or French (copies are available from ASAC 29, BD Gambetta, 7300 Chambery, France).

Dr. Hamer found that depending on the nature of the emotional shock or conflict different cancers would result. Fear of death can induce lung cancer; conflict between mother and children can induce cancer of the left breast; other conflicts can induce cancer of the right breast. Conflict over territory in the workplace can induce cancer of the colon. Repressed anger and bitterness can induce liver cancer. A loss of sense of worth due to a change in job status can induce bone cancer. Conflict with close family members can induce cancer of the stomach. Trauma involving water can induce cancer of the kidney. The following are a few examples: a few years ago I met a female cancer patient in France. She had cancer in both breasts which metastesized throughout the body. I asked her whether six months before the onset she experienced any traumatic event. She responded in the affirmative. Six months before the onset, all three sons had difficulty, one attempted suicide, another had an explosion in the house and the third one also had some problem. Then she had a big fight with her husband. It was soon after that she discovered cancer in both breasts and throughout the body. This case illustrates how a series of shocks brought about the cancer. Here are two more cases from Dr. Hamer's book: a mother had learned of her child taking drugs. This caused a conflict in her. She was concerned about the child and worried the father would find out and punish the child. This inner conflict caused her to develop cancer of the left breast. Later due to a change in business, the father moved away, thereby removing the conflict, and the illness ceased. Another case involved a child asking the mother to wash his feet because he thought they were dirty. The mother refused and the child climbed on top of a wash basin in an attempt to clean himself. He fell and hurt himself badly. The mother carried the guilt for having caused that for a long time. Later the mother came down with cancer of the kidneys. This conflict had something to do with water.

Dr. Hamer has found in recent years that not only cancer but all illnesses have connections with the emotions. If one has the opportunity to talk about one's problem and find a specific solution, that relieves the psychological stress. Once the emotional knots are untied, the brain lesion in turn reverses. In the healing phase one may have edema in the brain and fever. It is critical to avoid alcohol, tea or coffee. They can cause life-threatening situations.

More than ten years ago when I first started work at The University of Texas Cancer Center I met Dean Ornish, a medical student from the Baylor College of Medicine. He had just completed a study in which he gathered about twenty people with serious heart problems, teaching them how to meditate, do yoga and eat a vegetarian diet. They experienced significant improvement in their health. Some who had been on pain medication for over ten years did not need it anymore. Their heart condition improved.

From that first experiment Dr. Ornish later published a best-selling book, introducing in detail his program for reversal of heart diseases (Dr. Dean Ornish's Program for Reversing Heart Disease). His methods are open-heartedness and vegetarian food. Those with friends and warm families usually recover faster than those who are alone. He reported studies showing that warmth and affection can help prevent sickness. One study indicated those who are involved in charity work tend to live longer. Another interesting study involved rabbits fed a high cholesterol diet. Surprisingly those rabbits caged in the lower cages did not develop hardening of the arteries, while those in the higher cages did. Later it was found the technician looking after the rabbits was of short stature. After feeding the rabbits she would play with the ones in the lower cages. The rabbits housed in the high cages did not get any attention. Not only humans need affection, but animals as well.

Dr. Ornish's work has received recognition in the medical field. To make vegetarian food tasty, he invited some well known chefs to create many tasty vegetarian recipes. He also teaches ways to open one's heart, improving communications between people and within oneself. In communication he suggested that if one expresses one's feelings and not criticisms, it will improve relationships. Expressing one's feelings, whether positive or negative, will shorten the distance between people. For example one can say "I feel angry, happy or sad, etc." If one says instead, "You should not do this and that," then the other person will feel attacked and might respond negatively, inviting conflict. This would block the communication. To improve one's inner communication, yoga and meditation are suggested.

I have presented information on the relationship between open-heartedness and health from Eastern and Western sources. Now we will probe further the reason why open-heartedness is the wellspring of longevity and good fortune.

From Chinese phrases, we can learn about the right way of living. For example, "harmony generates prosperity," "charitable families will have much to celebrate," "planting squash begets squash, planting beans begets beans," "virtue brings good reward, evil brings negative results," "helping others is the root of happiness." We will come to the same conclusion from observing nature: seeds of sweet melon will produce sweet melons, and seeds of bitter melon will produce bitter melons. One never hears of planting a banana tree and harvesting apples. The law of the universe is that of a circle, whatever is sent out comes back to us. If we have an open heart, not harming others and are loving, we are going to be smiling and happy. Whatever we wish, whether it is health, happiness, longevity and even wealth will be ours.

There is a popular book written five hundred years ago in the Ming Dynasty entitled, "Liao-Fan's Four Lessons" or "How to Change Your Destiny." Why is this book still popular after five hundred years? The book described real life experiences of Mr. Yuan Liao Fan, and how he changed his whole life through application of the univeral law (the law of the circle). Others later following these principles also changed their lives. "Liao Fan's Four Lessons" was written from a father to son, filled with warmth and fully reflecting the love and caring of a father. Yuan Liao-Fan was a well respected magistrate in the Ming Dynasty. His four lessons are: The principle of fate, the method of repentance, the method of accumulating merit, and the benefit of humility. The book described in brief how Mr. Yuan lost his father at an early age. His mother urged him to study medicine. Later he met an astrologer, Mr. Kung, who told him that according to his horoscope he had the opportunity to study and receive official positions. He should study in order to pass government examinations instead. In the period of twenty years, his life unfolded as predicted by Mr. Kung. He thought that if all is fate, then what is the use of wishing for anything. He lost interest in studying and started to meditate. Once while meditating for three days and three nights with a Zen master in Nanjing, he realized that destiny can be changed by proper understanding. In his horoscope he was not to have a son, and he would not pass the highest level of imperial examination. Because he learned to repent and accumulate positive energy, he completely changed his life. "Liao-Fan's Four Lessons" is worthy of reading (see appendix for the English translation).

When the heart is open, one is open-hearted and happy. Health and good fortune naturally follow.

July 1991, Denver

Chapter 2
The Basic Cause of Open-Heartedness - Not Harming Others

There is a Chinese saying: "If you do not commit regretable deeds, there is no fear of ghosts knocking at your door at midnight." If one does not harm others, then one will have peace of mind. This is the basic cause of happiness. There are five guidelines for not harming others: not killing, not stealing, not engaging in sexual misconduct, and abstaining from alcohol and intoxicants. The following are brief explanation for each.

Do Not Kill: All life forms, whether human, animals and insects desire life and fear death. We celebrate the birth of new life and run away from dead bodies. People look forward to spring and when autumn comes with leaves falling, there is a sense of melancholy. If we wish for health, happiness, peace and longevity, we need to protect life. We need to avoid killing, directly or indirectly. In Chinese, there is a saying: "If you wish to know the cause of wars and conflicts in the world, listen to the midnight cries at the slaughter house." If we kill, we naturally plant the seeds of short life and much sickness. Remember that the universe is a big circle; what goes around comes around. There are other folk sayings in China: "Eating vegetables and tofu will keep you in peace." In this simple phrase is profound wisdom. There is now much medical evidence that vegetables and whole grains can help prevent many chronic illnesses, such as cancer, heart diseases, diabetes, etc. An additional benefit of not killing is that one will have a fine demeanor, kind and loving, and will be liked by others. Think of the murderers in prison. Each one of them looks mean and frightening. To have happiness one must not kill.

Do Not Steal: Everyone cherishes their own personal belongings. If they are lost, stolen or robbed, one would be quite upset. "Do unto others what one wishes oneself." "Do not steal" includes not generating wealth unethically. The benefit of not stealing is that one will not be lacking in material wealth.

Do Not Lie: "Trouble comes out of the mouth, sickness comes through the mouth." In speech we can easily say something that we regret later. If we are honest, we can have the trust of others. This will help in long lasting friendship and harmony at home. Those who habitually lie become so confused themselves that they cannot distinguish reality from imagination. Lying harms oneself and others. How can one be happy, then? "Do not lie" includes not telling little white lies and giving insincere flattery. They are not harmless.

Do Not Engage in Sexual Misconduct: Simply put, do not engage in relations outside of a normal relation between a man and a woman. Traditionally sexual misconduct denotes any relationship other than that between husband and wife. These days many people have relations before marriage and therefore the modification of the definition. The intimate relationship between a man and a woman is the most complex in the world. It can be heaven or hell, a happy story or a tragedy. Because the impulse for possesiveness is very strong in an intimate relationship, monogomy is important to happiness. If a third person gets involved in this intimate relationship, it is bound to bring sadness. It may cause one to lie or to commit drastic actions such as killing. How could one be happy under such circumstances?

Abstain from Alcohol and Intoxicants: Alcohol can alter our mind. Under the influence of alcohol one can lose good judgement. A person may normally be rational, but because of alcohol, they can kill, steal, lie, and engage in sexual misconduct. If one wishes to be open-hearted (happy), it is best not to drink.

Chapter 3
Removing the Obstruction to Open-heartedness

After mastering the basic course to open-heartedness, then one can work on removing the obstructions to open-heartedness. First, one must REPENT PAST HARMFUL ACTIONS TO OTHERS AND ONESELF: The analogy is like being bitten by a poisonous snake; one must suck out the poison, then apply medication. In addition to repenting wrong doing, one should make the determination not to repeat the wrongful action. The most effective way to repent is to do so in front of elders or the victim. It that is not possible, visualize them in front of you or in front of Buddhas and Bodhisattvas, then repent.

FORGIVE ONESELF AND OTHERS: After repentance, then we should let go of the burden, forgive oneself and others. There is no need to dwell on it. If others have harmed us, by not forgiving, everytime we think of the person, we are harmed again.

TRANSFORM ANGER AND HATRED WITH PATIENCE: Anger and hatred are the major obstructions to open-heartedness. To transform them with patience does not mean repressing the emotions, but with mind transformation, to change the blind reaction. From the perspective of the law of the universe, hatred can only harm us. Whatever is sent out comes back to us eventually. Patience does not mean that we allow

13

others to chop us up like vegetables or let others take advantage of us. Most importantly it is not to be upset, and angry, but calmly think about the best way to handle the situation. When we are filled with anger, our ability to think is significantly decreased. Blind reaction is like adding fuel to the fire; it will merely worsen the situation. When we are faced with people who are child-like and unreasonable, we can treat them like sick children running a high fever., There no need for anger.

TRANSFORM MISERLINESS WITH GENEROSITY: Generous people have many friends. A miser is sure to be lonely. To be happy and open-hearted, one has to give, especially to those that need us. "Helping others is the source of happiness," when we are generously helping others, we will be very happy.

TRANSFORM ARROGANCE WITH GRATITUDE: There is a common saying: "Contentment keeps one happy." But when arrogance dominates, then one is dissatisfied and blames God and others. Discontentment brings unhappiness. Gratitude can change arrogance and discontentment. Often when one is in good graces, one does not realize it. Everyday the sun rises, and the rain comes at the right time; we do not notice. If we have too little or too much rain, then we appreciate the times when the weather was good. If one day the sun were gone, we would all die for sure. We should have this feeling of gratitude all the time, happily thanking Heaven and Earth. We have much to be thankful in our life: friends and relatives, father and mother, children, health. As along as we are alive we have the opportunity to create our lives. Just as the saying goes: "As along as the green mountain is there, no need to worry for fire wood."

TRANSFORM JEALOUSY WITH REJOICING: To get the red eye when we see the success of others makes us most unhappy. The best treatment for "red-eye disease" is rejoicing, feeling happy for others success and good deeds. When we rejoice, not only we are happy but also plant the seeds of our success.

TRANSFORM ATTACHMENT WITH EQUANIMITY: "Equanimity" means to eliminate strong feelings of like and dislike. Ordinarily we are loving and happy with our own family and good friends. If we are separated from them then we become very unhappy. Actually with an open heart we meet "families" everywhere, then we are happy all the time. To meet is to have connection.

The above are several methods to remove obstructions to open-heartedness. If one can do it, then one can be happy.

Chapter 4
Meditation - Training
in Equanimity

Sue Dong Po, the great poet and scholar from the Sung dynasty once proudly wrote the following:

Bowing down to the Heaven among Heavens,
Radiating Lights filling the thousand worlds,
Unmoved by the eight worldly winds,
Sitting in the midst of the purple gold lotus.

The poem describes the exalted state of an enlightened being, He sent this poem, which hinted that his spiritual attainment was like that of the enlightened being, to his good friend, a zen master across the river. His friend, after reading it, simply replied on the back: "Eructation." Sue Dong Po was enraged when he saw that and rushed over to argue with him. He found the door shut with a note on the door: "Unmoved by the eight worldly winds, but sent across the river by one eructation."

What are the eight worldly winds: gain, loss, praise, criticism, happiness, pain, fame, and obscurity. Usually we are blown about by these eight worldly winds. Without self-mastery, how can one be calm and equanimous? Usually we react to pleasant things with attachment and to unpleasant things with aversion. Otherwise one is in this numb state. Thoughts constantly rise and fall, with not a moment of peace. In order to believe this, just observe one's breath upon inhalation and exhalation to see if one can be calm. Breathing is very simply air going in and out of the nostrils. If we observe the breath, we will notice that our mind is constantly fluttering from worrying about this and that, or from dissatisfaction with this and that. This mental stress is a tremendous burden on the body, exhausting a lot of energy. If we can control our thoughts then we can significantly improve the health of our body and mind and even our life. All that we do begins with a thought. If the thoughts are changed, of course the behavior is changed and our life is improved.

Taming the mind is like taming a wild horse. One must be patient and persistent. It is important not to rush it, or the mind can rebel. Because of the close connection between body and mind, relaxing the body will help relax the mind. Sit in a chair with the back slightly forward. Right foot over left foot at the ankle. Relax the forehead, eye-brow, and corners of the mouth. Then relax the muscles behind the knees and heels. With palms together rest them on the lap. Watch the breath, in and out. If the mind is too excited then watch the exhalation. If the mind is too drowsy, then watch the inhalation. If other thoughts come, let them come and go. In the beginning meditate like this for ten minutes, extending to thirty minutes. During other times of the day one can also remind oneself to watch the breath.

The activity of the brain is connected with breathing. When we are relaxed, the brain-wave is slower than our talking state. The breath is also slower. The reverse is also true. When we slow down the breath, the brain-wave also slows down, and our mind relaxes. When we are emotionally agitated, if we immediately slow down our breath, the emotions will relax. Deep breathing is a good method for taming the mind. Place the palms at the area below the navel. When exhaling, push in the palms, and extend the abdomen when inhaling, to the count of eight. Hold the breath for eight counts and exhale to the count of eight. Breathe naturally in between. After a few moments of deep breathing, the mind quiets down.

Chapter 5
Light and Sound Therapy

Light and sound can affect both our mind and our body, especially our Chi or life energy. It is said that most people use only 10% of their brain. Through the stimulation of light and sound therapy, it may be possible to tap into our hidden potential. Light and sound therapy can also help us express ourselves. When one is expressing oneself, one is most happy.

The sunlight after refraction will give the following colors: red, blue, yellow, green, orange, purple violet, and indigo. To use light or color to bring about positive changes, only bright colors are used. Every color has both a positive and a negative impact on us, depending on its clarity and luminosity. The brighter and clearer the color, the more positive the impact. The colors themselves have different effects on our mind. The practice of visualizing colored lights can stimulate our creativity and imagination. The following are the colors of light and the positive results which they produce:

Red: freedom, independence, leadership, pioneering spirit. It can be used to cut old patterns or habits that are no longer useful. Keep in mind what one wants to cut old patterns while visualizing red light at the same time. Sound: E

Sky Blue: patience, love, letting go. It can help communication between difficult relations. Sound: O

Yellow: joy, and organizational abilities. It can be used when unhappy. Sound: AH

Green: physical healing, growth and prosperity. Sound: A

Orange: self confidence, courage, and wisdom. Sound: AE

Purple Violet: healing at the emotional level, and inspiration, intuition. Sound: UU

Indigo: protection, oneness of all. Sound: OM

Practice with single color first. Look at a color, breathe in the color and make the corresponding sound. If one cannot visualize the color with eyes closed, open again to look at the color. With practice, one will improve. Visualizing color is actually involves recalling a memory of the color. Start with red to cut bad habits, but always heal with purple violet after the cut. Sky blue is very useful. Because it is love, it will help us forgive, and improve relations. In particular after the death of a loved one or the breakup of a romantic relationship, it is useful to send blue light to the unforgettable person. The light can come either from between the eye brows, or from the heart. Practice this for a few minutes everyday and one will notice a difference in one week. Sky blue light also can help in pain relief, even sleeping with a blue light bulb.

After one is familiar with visualizing a single color, one can do the following rainbow meditation: Visualize oneself at a meadow, with the green grass below and blue sky above. In front of oneself is a Mayan pyramid, flat on top and with many steps leading to the top. As you walk on to the first step, visualize oneself being filled with red light. At the second step, visualize blue light. Third step yellow light, fourth, green light, fifth, orange light, sixth, purple violet, seventh, indigo. When one reaches the top, take in the sun light, which has all the colors. Know that you can come up any time for recharge. For now, return by stepping down one step and visualizing indigo light, then purple violet, orange, green, yellow, blue, and red. Return to your place of sitting and open your eyes.

The practice of sound can also start with a single sound, like a rainbow E, O, Ah, A, AE, UU, OM all in one breath. Sound can change one's mind and Chi in the same way light can. The power of mantras are based on this principal. The mantra for compassion OM MANI PADME HUM is very beneficial for opening the heart. Recite it often.

People often ask me if there are books in which they can read more about the sound and light therapy that I teach. My answer is that I did not learn it from a book and therefore cannot recommend any. My meditation teacher in Houston, Liane Crawford, has very special gifts and taught me all that I know about light and sound. For myself, within six months of practicing, I went through some major changes. For years I would wear only green and blue, never red or orange, or yellow. I was also quite shy and introverted. After only a short time of working with the different colors, I started to wear bright orange, yellow, etc. Pretty soon my wardrobe was like that of the rainbow itself. I also found it easier to express myself, and happier, too. Since then I have had the opportunity to share the system with others and saw their transformation. Sky blue is useful for harmony and healing emotional wounds. I have seen it work again and again. Even lighting a blue light bulb in the family dining room helped one family to have more harmony and conversation instead of fighting.

In China there is a long tradition of blessing water with mantras such as Om Mani Padme Hum for healing purposes. As one recites the mantra, visualize light pouring into the glass of jar of water, blessing it to remove all sickness and obstacles.

Even today there continue to be stories of people being healed through drinking mantra-blessed water and reciting mantra. Just think, we are made up mostly of water. Just as the vibration of the mantra can change water, so can it change our body and mind.

Chapter 6
Chi Gong

The term Chi Gong covers Wu-Shu or martial arts, meditation, and the form that combines both movement and meditation for healing. The Chi or life energy with which Chi Gong works, affects both the mind and the body. Besides helping to harmonize the body, it is very useful for balancing the emotions.

In 1981 I first encountered Chi Gong in the parks of Beijing. I remember people with serious illnesses (for example, cancer patients) who were practicing Chi Gong. They were quite lighthearted. It was only after returning to the U.S., and through introducing Chi Gong, that I realized how useful it is for balancing emotions. American students practicing Chi Gong release a lot of repressed emotions, including sadness, anger and fear. After these are released, one naturally is happy. Of course Chi Gong's effect is not limited to balancing emotions. When the life energy is balanced, the body also becomes healthy.

There are at least one hundred forms of Chi Gong. It is best to find a good teacher with whom to study. A very simple form is introduced here; it comes from the preliminary form in Waidangong:

Stand with feet parallel to the shoulders. Relax the muscles behind the knees. Bring in the stomach and tighten the muscles around the rectum. Look straight ahead and allow the hands to drop on both sides. Relax the whole body and raise the index fingers. If one has practiced other forms of Chi Gong, the arms will start to vibrate spontaneously. Otherwise, move the wrists up and down in imitation. Start with ten minutes, slowly increase to thirty minutes. After practice, avoid drinking cold water, contacting cold air or washing. Allow at least 15 to 30 minutes before eating. For stroke patients, someone can help move the paralyzed arm in the same way. Some have regained the normal functioning of the paralyzed side. Others have shrunk their tumors (please refer to "Cancer Patients Exercising Their Way Back To Health for more information").

Denver, July, 1991.

Chinese Patients Exercise
Their Way Back To Health
(originally published in
East West Journal, March 1983)

My introduction to Chi gong, an ancient Chinese system of therapeutic exercises which is largely unknown to the West, took place about one week after my arrival in Beijing in September of 1981. Under the auspices of the National Academy of Sciences (Committee for Scholarly Communication with the People's Republic of China) I was to spend three months at the Cancer Institute in Beijing (Peking) collaborating with their scientists on a project studying the modifying effect of a regional Chinese diet on the incidence of esophageal cancer.

It was the first morning after settling into the National Labor Union Guest House, which was to be my home for the next three months. Suffering from jet lag, I woke up hours before having to report to work at the Cancer Institute, located just around the corner. I decided to go for a walk in the park across the street. Once outside, I was confronted with a continuous stream of bicyclists. The traffic, even at this hour, was unlike anything that I had ever seen. There were at least three lanes of bicycles going in each direction. I looked across the street to the entrance of Ritan Park and was bewildered. Suddenly I remembered my cousin's advice on crossing the streets in China: "Just walk at a normal pace. Don't stop or slow down and the bicycles will go around you." I stepped off the curb and walked with my eyes focused directly ahead of me. To my amazement, I found myself on the other side of the street, at the gateway to a totally new experience.

Ritan Park, located only a few blocks away from the American Embassy, was once an imperial ceremonial ground known as the Sun Temple. A burst of flowers in bright red, orange, and yellow greets visitors at each of the four entrances. The spacious grounds of the park, dotted with evergreens, surround a small hill with a pagoda on top and several buildings. A pond with fountains and a sculpture of flying swans completes the imperial scene. In the center is the temple itself, an enclosure surrounded by a circle of walls. In the imperial days, all of this was off-limits to ordinary people, but now it is open to the public.

In the early morning hours the park bustles with activity. Men with weathered faces sit on a bench deeply engrossed in a lively conversation. They stop now and then to admire the cages of birds resting at their feet. A short distance away more bird-cages hang from the trees while their owners stroll nearby keeping a watchful eye on them. A young couple giggles while playing badminton, and joggers pass by. Hidden voices sing an aria from a famous Western opera.

In the shadows of pine trees several groups of people perform various slow movements. A banner next to one group reads "Beijing Athletic Association, Tai Chi Chuan." Another reads "Beijing Chi Gong Research Association." I move closer to the Chi Gong group, because I had heard of the recent popularity of this ancient healing art. A robust woman in a blue jacket and baggy blue pants leads the group: "*Xi-xi, hu; xi-xi, hu* [*Xi* means inhale, and *hu* means exhale]." The breathing drill is synchronized with the steps of a slow walk. "Relax, swing your arms to the left, to the right." The students appear to be totally absorbed with their walk, eyes half-closed, oblivious to others around them.

The Chi Gong classes, which start at six a.m. and last an hour, attract people with various chronic illnesses. The Chinese believe that Chi Gong can combat a host of ailments including diabetes, heart disease, arthritis, liver and kidney problems, and cancer. Hospital patients have found that by doing Chi

Gong exercises every morning the side-effects of cancer treatments are reduced. They notice improved appetite and sleep, as well as an increase in overall immune resistance. And best of all, they become optimistic and cheerful. This is no small feat because cancer is such a psychologically devastating disease. Chi Gong deals directly with the psychological needs of cancer patients, a virtually unexplored area in modern Western medicine.

As a cancer researcher, I was particularly interested in the Chi Gong class for cancer patients. When I inquired about signing up for the classes, a bystander directed me to Mr. Fu, the person in charge of registration. "What is your illness? Do you have a doctor's diagnosis?" he asked. I explained that I was just interested in learning the exercises for cancer patients because I work in cancer research. He shook his head and said: "The exercises can be practiced only by cancer patients. Besides, foreign guests cannot resigter without special permission from the secretariat of the Chi Gong Research Association." I was surprised that he knew I was not local. Because I was born in Taiwan but had ancestral roots in Hunan, I spoke fluent Chinese. I even had on a blue jacket and baggy blue pants and was trying my best to blend in.

I pressed for an explanation. "Oh, it is easy. The way you move and your facial expressions give you away," he said. When I asked further about the success of the Chi Gong class for cancer patients, Mr. Fu said: "Let me put it this way, in the one-and-a-half years since the beginning of the classes, we have never heard of one single case where the patient came one day and did not make it the next." Our conversation was interrupted when a man came up to register his wife, who had cancer. I was not really satisfied with Mr. Fu's remarks but they were intriguing. All he said was that patients who can come to the class do not die the very next day. It told nothing of their condition after they stopped coming to class or how the exercises had helped them.

My early morning walk became a daily ritual. I learned more about Chi Gong. "Before you start the exercise, imagine a happy event. Let that image totally engulf you. Pick a stationary object in your mind. Focus on it. If you have high blood pressure, choose a low-lying object like a small flower. If your blood pressure is low, choose an object at eye level like a small pine tree. Return to the image when distracting thoughts interfere with your concentration. Don't concentrate too hard either."

I also learned that many of the students in the cancer class were patients at Ritan Hospital across the street. They claimed the daily one to two hours of Chi Gong exercises contributed significantly to their fight against cancer. At the very least it seemed to reduce the side-effects of cancer treatments, such as loss of appetite, weight loss, and lowering of white blood cell counts. Improved appetite and sleep are usually the first noticeable changes. "I was very depressed at first," a woman athlete in her thirties told me in speaking about her cancer. "But after I came here, and saw how cheerful everyone else was, I stopped worrying." Indeed the most striking feature of the Chi Gong classes is the optimism and cheerfulness of the students.

It is well known that two of the side-effects of cancer are depression and fear. Chi Gong deals directly with the psychological aspect of the disease. Even before the cancer patients begin the program, their confidence is bolstered by the positive experience of more advanced students of Chi Gong. In addition, as part of the Chi Gong exercises, the patient's mind is focused on pleasant images or memories. All of this creates a positive mental attitude in the patient. To what extent this may contribute to the benefit of Chi Gong is largely unknown since the psychological aspect of cancer is still not fully understood. Scientific studies have shown that stress can stimulate the neuroendocrine system, leading to depression of the immune system. Furthermore, the genesis and growth of cancer can be influenced by stress through such mechanisms. Removal of psychological stress alone can alter the neuroimmunal functioning of the body to the extent that it can change the course of cancer development.

Ritan Hospital is the best known cancer hospital in the country. It has all the facilities of a modern hospital including surgery, radiation, and chemotherapy. The only Chinese touch is the presence of an herbal pharmacy from which doctors can order traditional herbals to counteract the side-effects of the Western treatments on their patients. In the hospital courtyard, gowned patients walk or sit on the benches in order to enjoy the autumn sun. On a typical afternoon most of the hospital rooms remain empty because patients go to the courtyard or to the park across the street.

Patients are expected to look after themselves. As long as they are physically capable, patients make their own beds and pick up their own meals from the meal carts that come to their wards. The meals are ordered ahead of time and an array of typical Chinese dishes is offered. Those who are taking Chi Gong classes rise early and after changing into street clothes arrive in the park for their daily Chi Gong exercises. Classes always finish in time for them to return to the hospital for breakfast.

Many of the hospital personnel are ambivalent toward the classes. "It just does not look good when our patients run around in the park," a head nurse was told by her superior. "But the patients complain that the hospital gate opens at six a.m. instead of five-thirty a.m." Apparently the gate opens later as winter approaches. The physicians and nurses agree that patients taking Chi Gong classes appear not to suffer from the side-effects of the radiation and chemotherapy treatments.

They continue eating well and maintain their weight. One study performed at the Beijing Lung Cancer Research Institute showed that Chi Gong exercises increased immune resistance among lung cancer patients. This was indicated by studies of white blood cell counts and skin tests. Some physicians recommend Chi Gong to their patients as a last resort when other therapies fail.

In order to fully appreciate the value of Chi Gong it is necessary to consider it in the context of the philosophical foundation of Chinese medicine. Chinese medicine views a human as an integral composite of mind, emotions, and body which are intimately connected with the heavenly and earthly environments. Health and longevity result from harmonizing these components within oneself and in the environment. This requires following the seasonal changes in the choice of foods, seasonal fluctuations in sleeping and walking patterns, and temperance in all indulgences. Most importantly, a tranquil mind, which is achieved through reducing desires and quieting random thoughts, is essential in maintaining health.

Illnesses are perceived as the results of imbalances in any of these aspects of living. Emotional stresses can induce physical problems while physical problems can induce emotional responses. For example, worry and anxiety are related to the heart, and continual worry or excessive anxieties can result in heart problems. Anger and the liver are related. While angry emotions can injure the liver, liver problems can also bring on frequent outbursts of anger or an attack of bile as they say in the West. The psychosomatic aspect of health and disease has an important place in the tradition of Chinese medicine. The interrelationship between the physical and emotional states has guided medicine in China for thousands of years.

The term *Chi Gong* is difficult to translate. Firstly, chi has the meanings of air, breath, or gas. It is the substance traditionally believed to permeate the human body, flowing along paths called meridians. These meridians are not linked to the vascular system but influence metabolism and the functioning of different parts of the body. This Chinese view of the human body with chi flowing through the meridians is still somewhat of a mystery. When the flow of chi is unobstructed, health prevails. Obstruction of chi in any part of the body brings on sickness. Obstruction can be brought on through neglect and abuse of the body or from emotional disturbances. All the traditional Chinese medical practices work on removing obstructions. The flow of chi can be manipulated by inserting needles at specific points on the meridians and this is of course the new popular practice of acupuncture. To illustrate how pervasive this concept of chi is in Chinese culture, the Chinese word for anger is *shen-chi* or "(to) generate chi" and the word for temperament is *pe-chi* or "spleen chi." Even the word for weather, *tian-chi,* means "heavenly chi".

Secondly, gong means work, effort, or accomplishment. Together the two words Chi Gong mean "working on the chi" or "mastery of the chi." This mastery of chi is accomplished through specific movements, rhythmic breathing, sounds, and mental imagery. The most famous of Chi Gong movements imitate the movements of five animals: bear, tiger, monkey, deer, and bird. The breathing accompanying the movements are generally slow and unhurried and perhaps softly audible. Depending on the nature of the disease, the rhythm may be two short inhalations, one exhalation, or one in and one out. The emphasis for cancer patients is on breathing in a lot of oxygen and the two short inhalations and one exhalation method of breathing is preferred.

However, the essential aspect of Chi Gong has to do with the mind. The success of Chi Gong depends to a large degree on whether the mind is relaxed during the exercises. To arrive at the mental state of tranquility and peacefulness, students of Chi

Gong are first advised to avoid indulging in the seven emotions: elation, fear, fright, sadness, yearning, anger, and worry. Excesses in any of these emotions prevent reaching the state of tranquility and aggravate any existing health problems. Furthermore, interference by random thoughts during exercising is prevented by focusing on certain themes—imagery of objects or words. Chi Gong exercises often employ only imagery to guide the flow of Chi to different parts of the body. Whether the unobstructed flow of Chi is accomplished through movements, breathing, sound, or imagery, the end result is an improvement in health and longevity.

The earliest mention of Chi Gong was recorded in the classic of internal medicine, the *Nei Ching,* over four thousand years ago. *Nei Ching,* or more fully *Huang Ti Nei Ching,* is the oldest known writing on Chinese medicine. It provides the foundation for the practice of Chinese medicine. Also during recent archaeological excavations of Han Tombs in Changsha, Hunan, which are approximately two thousand years old, archaeologists found among medical writings extensive drawings of Chi Gong movements, indicating that even in the Han dynasty it was still popular as a form of therapy.

The practice of Chi Gong, however, is not restricted to the context of medicine. Until very recently it was particularly popular among Taoists, who strive to follow the Tao or the order of the Universe. They felt that by being in harmony with nature one enjoys not only peacefulness of mind but also longevity and a youthful body. The practice of Chi Gong is consistent with the attainment of inner harmony. Since Taoists preferred secluded areas far away from civilization to practice their beliefs, it was necessary for them to learn self-defense to protect themselves from wild animals and bandits. One school of Chi Gong developed into the marital arts. In time Chi Gong became associated with the exhibition of unusual powers: crushing bricks with bare fists, jumping over high walls, immobilizing an enemy with the touch of a finger. This approach was practiced only by small groups of people and considered too esoteric for the general public.

Today large numbers of Chinese are turning to Chi Gong for health reasons. According to the Chi Gong Research Association, which sponsors many classes, over ten thousand people are enrolled throughout the greater Beijing area. In addition, organizations such as the Beijing Athletic Association sponsor their own Chi Gong classes. There are also classes personally supervised by the famous Chi Gong master, Madame Guo Lin in Ditan (Earth Temple) Park and the Purple Bamboo Garden.

Madame Guo first taught Chi Gong in the parks more than ten years ago, long before the current popularity. She is the one individual most responsible for the current interest in Chi Gong. Even now, at the age of 73, she still personally supervises classes. On Sunday mornings she can be seen working with her thirty or so volunteer teachers and aides at Ditan Park, and on Monday and Wednesday mornings she teaches at the Purple Bamboo Garden park.

Guo Lin does Chinese brush-paintings of landscapes and flowers for a living and is a founding member of the Beijing Art Institute. She has been painting since she was eight, but she has an even longer experience with Chi Gong. Brought up mostly by her grandfather, a Taoist, she was first instructed in the ancient exercises of Chi Gong when she was six. Later, in her career as a landscape painter, she found herself visiting many famous mountains of China, where she encountered several Chi Gong masters, with whom she studied.

She modified Chi Gong specifically to cure diseases after her own bout with cancer thirty years ago. It was during the stressful years of the "liberation" of Shanghai that she developed cancer of the uterus. After six operations to stop the spread of the cancer she started working on modifying Chi Gong to restore her health. It worked and now she has been practicing the "new" Chi Gong for over twenty years and teaching it for over ten years. She has now turned over teaching responsibilities to many of her former students. She serves as a consultant to the Chinese Chi Gong Research Association and personally supervises only the more difficult cases. In Beijing alone there are three to four hundred students who participate in her classes annually.

The popularity of her classes was helped by numerous newspaper reports as well as several television documentaries about Chi Gong. She and her assistants have been invited to start classes all over China. A story in an important Chinese scientific magazine drew many inquiries from readers. In response to the intense interest generated by the article, the magazine asked Guo Lin to write books about Chi Gong, which resulted in two titles (available only in China). The first, *New Chi Gong Therapy for Beginners,* describes the basic exercises for treating chronic illnesses. The second book, *New Chi Gong Therapy for Cancer,* is more specific. In addition to basic exercises it describes special ones geared for cancer patients. In both books there are many illustrations depicting the exercises in great detail.

The case histories at the end of the books contain hospital records as well as the patients' own accounts of the disease. In the first book, the cases include chronic heart problems, hepatitis, digestive problems, kidney inflammation, arthritis, glaucoma, and respiratory problems. All were cleared up after several months of practice. Hospital checkups showed healthy patients free of the original problems. Mme. Guo Lin's second book covers many types of cancers including lung, breast, liver, and lymph node. In almost all cases the disease had progressed to the late stage with extensive metastasis. Here are two interesting cases:

Mr. Gau, age 55. Profession: Assistant Secretary in the Department of the Navy. In 1976, Gau was diagnosed from x-rays and a biopsy as having cancer of the lung. Exploratory surgery revealed extensive metastasis. The doctors closed his chest without any further surgical operation. He received radiation and chemotherapy treatments as well as herbal medicine. Despite all these efforts his health continued to deteriorate. He suffered from swelling of the lower limbs after the chemotherapy treatment as well as headaches, dizziness, poor appetite and poor sleep. His white blood cell count fell below 4600 compared to an average of 9000. His doctors guessed he had six months to live.

In May of 1977 he was introduced to Chi Gong. In the beginning he could do only very limited exercises, walking no more than two hundred steps per day. Gradually he did more— three hundred, four hundred, and eventually ten thousand steps each day. This is the level he has maintained for the last four years. Like most new students of Chi Gong he was skeptical at first but after two weeks he noticed improvements: better sleep at night, bigger appetite. The swelling in the lower limbs also slowly went away as well as his radiation-induced pneumonia. After the first year he went back for a checkup. His doctor was amazed that Gau was still alive. Two years later he went for another checkup—the doctor was even more surprised. Three years later his annual checkup indicated that he was in good health. Gau returned to work in March of 1980 and except for his daily "walks" leads a normal life. When I met him in Madame Guo's art studio in November of 1981, he was in good health.

Ms. Chiang, age 42. Profession: Research Assistant, Institute of Dynamics, Chinese Academy of Sciences. Chiang was first diagnosed in 1975 as having cancer of the right breast with involvement of the lymph gland in the left breast. In May of the same year the right breast was removed. In March of 1977 the cancer spread to the ovary. A second operation removed the ovary. She was also given radiation and chemotherapy treatments. She began the Chi Gong exercises in July of 1977. The cancer that had earlier spread to the left breast ceased growing. The side-effects experienced during radiation and chemotherapy treatments such as loss of appetite, poor sleep, and lassitude all disappeared. Her blood count also returned to normal. Her physician noticed that macrophages obtained from her had the capacity to attack cancer cells. She has since returned to work and shows no signs of cancer. Originally she was expected to live only six months. It has now been more than three years since she started Chi Gong. Her case has inspired other patients with cancer and chronic illnesses in her institute to take up Chi Gong. In response to the interest, special classes have been organized at her place of work.

There are many more cases like these two. Madame Guo has records of over 7,000 cancer cases from the Chi Gong classes throughout China. There are even more cases of people with chronic illnesses who have regained their health through practicing this ancient exercise.

How has the Chinese government responded to the popular interest in this ancient healing art? Basically not at all. After all, China has more pressing problems, with "modernization" having the highest priority. This in part explains the lack of interest on the part of the medical establishment in Chi Gong. The cancer researchers at the Cancer Institute are preoccupied with modernizing laboratory research such as bringing in new equipment and techniques but are unaware of the remarkable movements taking place across the street in Ritan Park. When asked specifically about what they thought of Chi Gong, the response ranged from complete ignorance to mild interest. At a time when the top leadership is urging modernizations, paying attention to an ancient healing art is probably viewed as a retrograde step. Regardless of what the government or scientists think, the present popular interest in Chi Gong is likely to continue. To those who are suffering from pains of human illnesses it is what works that matters, be it a twentieth-century invention or a four-thousand-year-old exercise.

Since my visit to China last year, Madame Guo's work has received more recognition in China. At least two more articles have appeared in print about her work, one in an English lan-guage magazine, Women of China. *The other article, "Cancer Does Not Mean Death," written by the famous Chinese writer Ke Yan, appeared in a Beijing literary magazine. It was based on the author's own encounter with cancer and Chi Gong.*

Part II

Natural Vegetarian Food is the Best Medicine

Natural Vegetarian Food is the Best Medicine

In total I have been a vegetarian for eighteen years. At the surface, being a vegetarian or meat-eater is a food choice and habit. Most people in society are meat eaters and only a few choose to be vegetarian. A vegetarian would find inconviences in social occasions, sometimes even awkward situations. After being a vegetarian for a long time, working in cancer research for ten years, and studying Buddhism in depth, I realize the choice of food affects a person's health, as well as war and peace. It also affects a person's spiritual growth. The choice of food is not merely limited to the stomach and mouth. The longer I have been a vegetarian, the more of the world I traveled, the more I rejoice in the good fortune of those who are vegetarians. A vegetarian not only can enjoy health and long life, avoid accidental death and conflicts of war, but also increase love, and the great compassion that will take one to liberation.

There is ample and clear medical and nutritional evidence showing that a diet based on plants contributes to health. If anyone disagrees, it is because his scientific knowledge is out of date. In the experience of myself, family and friends, the change to a vegetarian diet brings improvement in health. I lived in the Indian Himalayan mountains for six months on vegetables, fruits, grains, beans and sesames. Occassionally I would have yoghurt. There were no vitamin supplements, and no health foods, and very little oil. Compared to the time in America, I was

41

healthier and even gained a little weight. Eating a vegetarian diet that is natural, not overly seasoned, or made into imitation meat and duck, one's health will definitely improve. A vegetarian diet can prevent cancer, diabetes, heart diseases, high blood pressure, allergy and parasites.

All conscious beings are afraid of death. If those of us who eat meat were to make a trip to the slaughter house and witness where our meats come from, then many of us would change to a vegetarian diet. All of us have innate compassion. The struggle and suffering at the time of death is the same for all living creatures. Animals are like humans; they generate hatred at the time of being killed. These "souls" of the animals hang around looking for opportunities to take revenge. This is another reason why meat-eating brings sickness and short lives. Chicago is a major center for slaughtering of livestocks. Those with ESP have commented on the density of animal spirits hanging over the city, casting a dark gloom over the entire city. The crime rate in Chicago is also very high, all and all not a peaceful city. New Zealand is known for exportation of meat. According to some Tibetan Lamas, because of the killing, it was difficult to establish Buddhism. Even though they tried many times to establish Buddhist centers, it was difficult to continue. The karma of killing, if too heavy, will destroy the roots of compassion, easily disconnecting from the liberation path of Buddhism. On the contrary, those who switch from a meat-based diet to a vegetable-based diet will enjoy lightening of the heart. The reason is very simple: the spirits of the animals no long come to claim the debt.

In nature we observe herbivores are calm and peaceful. The meat-eaters are cruel and violent. One day when everyone on earth stops killing for food, the day of world peace will arrive. Even though we cannot expect everyone to be like that, if we ourselves become vegetarians, we will become disengaged from wars. We would be born in areas where the crops are abundant, rain is timely, and there is no war. Imagine if there are so many advantages to being a vegetarian, why not be one?

Everyone pursues happiness, good fortune, long life and health. This can be obtained easily. "Being a vegetarian" is a most precious golden key that can open the door to life's treasure house. I hope friends will value this golden key and not throw it away.

February 1988, Sarnath, India

Chapter 7
My Awakening

From my childhood experience with allergies, I learned of the intimate relationship between food and illness. I had a weak constitution. Often after eating seafoods such as shrimp, I would develop hives. The Chinese doctor said my weak liver accounted for the frequent sickness. The year I turned eight, the entire family moved to Michigan for two years. Food in America was quite different from the food eaten in Taiwan. For instance, food is bought once a week at the supermarket. In Taiwan Mom would shop daily at the local farmers' market. Not only ice cream, soft drinks and chocolate were added to the daily diet; we also had hot dogs and chicken legs quite often. Within six months of moving to the U.S., my problem with hives worsened significantly. The problem would occur at least once or several times a week. The next year a medical expert was consulted. The doctor after much testing told me I was allergic to milk, peanuts, dust, and molds. After two years in America we returned to Taiwan. In the first year, the hives were still frequent, then lessened. Four years later we returned to the United States. Again within six months the hives became serious. I started taking anti-histamine pills, which made me drowsy most of the time. Then I started taking allergy shots monthly, which controled the allergies. The testing again confirmed I was allergic to molds, dust, pollen, and milk. This routine of monthly allergy shots went on for two years.

During the first year in college I read the book by Norman Walker, M.D., "Raw Vegetable Juices." His theory was that most of the diseases are caused by lack of organic minerals, found in fresh vegetables and fruits. In Chinese cuisine, there is not a tradition of eating salads; usually everything is cooked. After reading this book, I came to understand that my hives are connected with the food I was eating. Thus began the food "revolution" at home.

The first step I took was to add a salad to every dinner, made of finely grated vegetables. They are made of celery, carrots, cabbage, etc. Mom's reaction was: this salad is like the feed given to the chickens in Taiwan. Next, I changed the white rice to brown rice. Now Mom's comments were: just like what the peasants used to eat.

I also stopped eating meats, fish, chicken, and all sweets such as ice cream. I also stopped going to the doctor's for allergy shots. The doctor warned me that my allergies would return. This was eighteen years ago. In the eighteen years, I have traveled throughout China, Europe, America, eating all kinds of different foods. The problem with hives have essentially been cured. Only once when traveling in Europe for ten days, I sampled all the sweets in each cities visited. After returning to my place of residence, I had hives for one week. This is my first awakening: food and illnesses are connected. Doctors and school do not necessarily have the answer.

My awakening directly affected the family's health, and indirectly that of my friends. In the beginning, mother did not completely support the food revolution. Mom had always had complete control over the kitchen. But in six months, she started to enjoy significant improvement in her health. She then not only fully practiced the natural way of eating but also enthusiastically introduced it to friends. Before the change in diet, Mom had many health problems. From her younger days she had taken much medicine and shots, therefore weakening her system. Hawaii is rather humid; she suffered from alleries, running nose and could not breath easily at night. She received two years of shots. She also had constipation, high blood pressure and frequent headaches. Her hair was like dry grass. Whenever she got busy, she would get a stomach ache. She had been hospitalized three times. The doctor said she had a tumor in the uterus, holes in the kidney, and a gap between her stomach and small intestine. She had to take tranquilizers, and raise the feet during sleep, but her health still suffered. After the change in diet, in a short time the constipation was relieved. The allergies cleared without shots, and her hair became shiny. Even after hard work, she no longer suffered from headaches and stomach aches. She started growing vegetables in the backyard, full of energy. Each time after a physical examination, the results were always the same. The nurse would comment her blood pressure is like that of a young person. One year after the change in diet, she discovered a lump in the breast, very painful. The doctor scheduled surgery one month later. We immediately checked through our books on natural healing. For one week Mom went on a fruit diet, and took epsom salt baths to stimulate the elimination through the skin. On the lump she applied a compress made of linseed oil and spirit of camphor. After one month, the lump was gone. The doctor was not happy for mother. He had said there was no other way. This increased further my confidence in natural healing. Food plays an important role. The younger sisters (five altogether) did not have many health problems to begin with. After the change, they did not even have the common cold. In the eighteen years, the whole family have enjoyed health without sickness. Mom is now in her sixties, works ten hours a day, growing vegetables, working on her pottery. She hikes with the younger generation, not showing much sign of aging at all.

Houston, 1987

Chapter 8
The Role of Diet in
Cancer Prevention

To many people, cancer is viewed with fear as an incurable disease. In this section, I hope to offer my knowledge and to correct this misunderstanding. Cancer is not incurable. It is treatable and preventable. My emphasis is on prevention. It is always more difficult and expensive to treat, but easy and inexpensive to prevent.

First of all let me mention that for ten years I worked at the University of Texas System Cancer Center, M.D. Anderson Hospital and Tumor Institute. In the U.S., it ranks in the top three among cancer centers. It's facilities are complete in treatment, education and research. I started to work there after receiving my doctorate degree from Massachusettes Institute of Technology in 1977. My field of study is physical chemistry, not biochemistry. Therefore my research has been in the area of biophysics, different from most of my colleagues. My perception is very much influenced by my training, perhaps making me more open to natural healing.

Depending on the location of the cancereous growth, it is given different names. Essentially, cancer is uncontrolled cell growth. It is often capable of establishing new sites of growth away from the primary site.

In the U.S., cancer ranks number two as a cause of death, second to heart disease. Lung cancer is most common, followed by cancer of the large intestine and breast. The incidence of lung cancer in the U.S. is on the increase, especially among women. This is due to the increasing number of women who smoke.

Americans are very afraid of cancer. The survival rate for lung cancer, based on five year survival is only ten percent. I want to emphasize again that there is no difference in survival between those receiving treatment and those receiving no treatment. Often people think cancer treatment in the U.S. is very advanced. This is incorrect. The five year survival rate for cancer of the large intestine and breast is fifty percent. For lymphoma and leukemia, the survival rate is only three percent. From these numbers, it is clear that Western medicine does not have the answer to cancer, otherwise the survival rates would not be so low. It is possible that the whole direction of research is wrong. Cancer is treated as a local disease, neglecting the systematic considerations, in particular the biophysical aspects.

That cancer is preventable is based on the following facts:

First, the incidence of the disease is different in different countries. This indicates that cancer is not inevitable but occurs in dependence on the environment.

Second, the incidence of cancer changes upon migration. For example, stomach cancer is common in Japan. The incidence of stomach cancer among Japanese immigrants to the U.S. changes with each successive generation. By the second and third generation, the incidence is the same as that of American natives. This indicates that cancer is not genetic. The fact that the incidence of cancer changes upon migration indicates that the disease is preventable.

Third, the incidence of cancer can change with time. For example, the incidence of stomach cancer in the U.S. has steadily declined for the last fifty years, without specific intervention.

However there has not been significant progress in treatment of the disease. It is due predominantly to changes in food and life style.

Fourth, with the identification of cancer causing substances, through reducing contamination by carcinogens, certain cancers can be prevented. It is known, for example, that aflatoxin can induce liver cancer. Nitrosamine, formed in the stomach during degestion of protein, can induce stomach cancer. If we can reduce these substances, then we can reduce cancer.

Fifth, the development of cancer can be reversed. Research findings show that the incidence of cancer among smokers is several times that of non-smokers. The incidence of lung cancer among those who have quit smoking for five or ten years is much reduced. This is because removing the outside irritant, smoke, allows the body to regain its original defences.

The above is a brief summary of the main points. Now more elaboration and specifice examples will be given.

1. The incidence of large intestine cancer in different countries: The incidence of large intestine cancer is most frequent in the West, especially in New Zealand, Australia, U.S. and Canada, and less frequent in Europe, while Asia and Africa have the lowest incidence (see chart). Because New Zealand and Australia are not heavily industralized, to blame the high incidence on environmental pollution is implausible. Rather it is probably due to the high consumption of meat in New Zealand and Australia. Meat consumption is less in Europe, thus in proportion to the incidence of large intestine cancer. Meat consumption in Japan is only 10% that of New Zealand, and the incidence of large intestine cancer is also lower. There is a direct correlation between meat consumption and incidence of cancer of the large instestine.

Increased fat consumption causes increased secretion of bile juice. Bile juice is further broken down in the intestine by bacteria forming carcinogenic compounds. This has been proven in animal studies. Also this bile by-product, when painted on animal skin, can also induce cancer.

Death in women due to Cancer of the large intestine

	per 10,000	meat intake per day
New Zealand	40	309 gram
Unites States	30	280 gram
Great Britain	20	197 gram
Japan	7	30 gram

2. Within the same country, the incidence of cancer is also different: Among American Seventh-Day Adventists, for example, the incidence of cancer is lower than the American average, especially for the digestive system. More than fifty percent of adventists are vegetarians. This is consistent with the observed relation between diet and cancer. Even in regard to cancer of the breast and reproductive organs, the incidence of cancer for Seventh-Day Adventists is only 70% of the national average. Diet and hormone secretion are related, and hormones can influence the formation of carcinogens.

3. The incidence of lung cancer is on the increase over the last 20 years. This is directly attributable to smoking. Since 1987, lung cancer has become the main cause of death for women with cancer, surpassing cancer of the large intestine and breast. Not smoking is the best prevention for cancer, and also saves money. Unfortunately, it is also a difficult habit to change.

4. Previously, the example of lowered incidence of stomach cancer among Japanese immigrants in U.S. illustrated that cancer incidence is influenced by the enviroment. On the other

hand these immigrants' incidence of cancer of the large intestine increased to that of the American population within three generations. The decline in the incidence of stomach cancer in the U.S. is thought to be due to the following two reasons: due to advances in agriculture and transportation, fresh vegetables and fruits are available year round. In the northern part of the U.S., fresh vegetables were not easily available in the past. Fresh vegetables and fruits are rich in vitamin C, which can prevent the formation of nitrosamine. Americans eat salads, while Chinese do not. This is one of the reasons why stomach cancer is more common among Chinese. The second reason is the use of refrigerators, which reduces the conversion of nitrite to nitrate in leftovers; nitrate is a component in the formation of nitrosamine.

5. The role played by diet in the incidence of breast cancer is due to the secretion of prolactin, which increases the risk factor of breast cancer. Blood level of prolactin is influenced by the amount of fat in the diet. Studies conducted by Dr. Ernst Wynder more than ten years ago, showed that four nurses ingesting Western style food showed peak levels of protactin around four a.m. in each 24 hour period. When they changed to a vegetarian diet, the prolactin level was reduced by 60%. This explains why Asian women get breast cancer less frequently than Western women. Their intake of fat is lower.

6. The ratio of potassium to sodium in the diet is less often reported in the medical journals. The level of potassium and sodium intake can affect the incidence of cancer. Sodium is abundant in salt and M.S.G., while potassium is abundant in vegetables and fruits. Dr. B. Jansson from the University of Texas M.D. Anderson Hospital and Tumor Institute discovered the link. Taking epidemiological data from over twenty countries, he found that the intake of potassium is inversely pro-

portional to the incidence of cancer. He also found that as one ages, potassium starts to leak from the cells. In normal cells, the ratio of potassium to sodium is often as high as ten. The ratio of potassium to sodium decreases in cells undergoing division. Cancer cells also have lowered ratio of potassium to sodium. When cells are damaged, potassium is leaked from the cells, and cells start to divide. As one ages the risk of getting cancer increases, in part due to lowered level of potassium in the cells. Furthermore, it was found that people with certain illnesses producing high potassium levels had a lower incidence of cancer. How did Dr. Jansson get interested in the ratio of potassium to sodium? He had noticed that Seneca County in New York State has an extremely low incidence of cancer of all types compared with neighboring counties. The residents take their water from Seneca lake, which contains about ten times higher potassium than neighboring lakes. In Iran there are certain areas that have very high incidence of esophagus cancer. People in those areas eat mostly bread. Usually salt is added to flour in the making of bread. Areas that have low incidences of esophagus cancer eat mostly rice. I do not know about Taiwan, but in the U.S. salt is added to bread, to improve flavor. Most people may not realize such a small difference in diet can make a big difference in cancer incidence. I have found in cultivating cells that if potassium is added to the growth media, the cells can become normal. The following is an example: mouse leukemic cells cannot produce haemoglobin. When potassium is raised ten times in the growth media, the cells are able to produce haemoglobin. This indicates that the ratio of potassium to sodium plays an important role in the development of cancer. Most of these data are not available to the public, because we are in the developmental phase of the studies.

7. The role played by the environment in influencing cancer: Let us look at the example of Linxian county in Henan province.

That county has one of the highest incidences of esophagus cancer. Esophagus cancer is ordinarily not common. Geographically it is located in the mountain range of Henan having poor soil, deficient in many minerals, such as copper and zinc. Locally grown vegetables contain low levels of vitamin C. Vitamin C has a protective effect against cancer. Another unusual feature of the area is that nine years out of ten are drought, resulting in a lack of food. The local residents use tree leaves or grass as food. To improve the flavor, the practice of pickling is common. Pickling does not use salt. Yam leaves or leaves from trees are placed in a large urn, filled with water from washing rice, and sealed for three months. By then the mixture is filled with mold, and is eaten with rice. The moldy water is also consumed. The moldy water and vegetables contain many carcinogens. It is customary to keep corn bread for two or three weeks until covered with mold. This is similar to eating of blue cheese in the West. Research studies found that when this moldy corn bread was fed to rats, the rats would get esophagus cancer. In summary, the causes of esophagus cancer are two-fold: monotonous diet, low in nutrition, with no legumes; and consumption of carcinogens.

8. Animal research showing the link between diet and cancer mentioned above was conducted more than fifty years ago. Calorie intake was found to influence the formation of cancer. Increased caloric intake also increased the incidence of cancer. It is the case with chemically induced skin cancer. With breast cancer, whether virally or chemically induced, the trend is the same: increased caloric intake increases incidence.

Another experiment involved food restriction and the onset of cancer in rats. The group on unrestricted diet had a higher incidence of cancer. The group on a restricted diet (at least ½ to ⅓ of normal) the incidence of cancer is reduced. The results are as follows:

sarcoma: cancer incidence of the restricted diet group
is one-fourth that of the unrestricted group.

breast cancer: cancer rate of the restricted diet group
is one-seventh that of the unrestricted group.

skin cancer: cancer rate of the restricted diet group is
one-fifth that of the unrestricted group.

In general, the group on a restricted diet appeared healthier and
lived longer.

The above results were obtained more than fifty years ago.
At the time because of a lack of epidemiological data, and the
lack of world-wide cancer data, the results were ignored. In
recent decades due to the development of epidemiological data
and the increase in cancer, these results have received renewed
interest and attention. This also stimulated much research in
the area of cancer and diet.

Below is a summary of the recommendation made by the
National Cancer Institute to the American public on how to
reduce the risk of cancer:

1. Reduce fat intake: Americans receive 40% of caloric intake
from fat. The recommendation is to reduce it to 30%. Actually
this is still considerably higher than the 10% intake for Japanese.
Because it is difficult to change diet, the conservative 30%
suggestion was made. Hopefully this would reduce the incidence of breast and large intestine cancer.

2. Eat more fresh vegetables, fruits and whole grains: These
foods contain protective factors, such as plant hormones, and
vitamin C. Before we discuss cancer causing agents, let us focus
on protective foods. The liver plays the important role of de-
toxification. Its function depends on a variety of mixed function
oxidases. Plant hormones stimulate the production of these
enzymes. In animal studies, if plants containing high levels of

plant hormones were given at the same time as carcinogens, cancer incidences were reduced. Plant hormones are most abundant in young shoots. Therefore it is beneficial if one consumes sprouts frequently. Vegetables such as cauliflower, cabbage, and brussels sprouts have high levels of plant hormones. Another character of plant hormones is that they are relatively heat insensitive, so even after cooking they are effective.

Fiber also has protective effects, by reducing the transient time of waste product in the large intestine. Fiber comes mostly from grains, bran, brown rice, etc. These also contains more minerals. In the U.S., the soil in the South contains more selenium, thus the lowered incidence of cancer in the south. People on a refined diet will not get enough minerals. The recommendation of eating more whole grains is very good. Legumes contain also a protective factor, proteas inhibitor. This is very good protection against chemically induced cancer. In animal studies, the group getting soy beans had a lower incidence of cancer than the group getting milk. This also in part explains the high incidence of esophagus cancer in Linxian county, which produces hardly any soy beans. In contrast, Fan county, located only four hours away, has a much lower incidence, because they grow and consume soy beans there, grinding the soy into flour to make bread. This is worth noting.

3. Avoid smoked meat or salt-cured food: In the process of making these, carcinogens are produced. If one must eat meat, one should eat fresh meat.

4. Avoid contamination by carcinogens: For example in grain storage, avoid the formation of aflatoxin. This is extremely potent. A small amount can induce cancer.

5. Continue to identify other carcinogens, to reduce the risk of cancer.

6. Reduce the use of cigarettes and alcohol: We can only say that smoking is the one of the main causative factor in lung cancer. We will not say everyone who smokes will get cancer. The facts are that 90% of people who get lung cancer smoke. The other factors may be pollution, etc. Smoking and alcohol are often inseparable. Alcohol is a good solvent, allowing better penetration of carcinogens into skin, increasing the risk of cancer. I want to emphasize this point, to encourage stopping of smoking and consumption of alcohol.

The above introduces many causative factors to cancer. What does one do after contracting cancer? It is rather late to be talking prevention, but at least the diet should be consistent with that for prevention, to save one's life. Cancer treatment diets are popular in the U.S. The anti-cancer diets are vegetable based, to reduce the ingestion of carcinogens. Most hospitals are just beginning research in this area, and not much has been done as yet. Let me emphasize the importance of the potassium/sodium ratio. I have mentioned before that in our research it was found that increasing the potassium level in the growth media can revert cancer cells to normal cells. The best potassium source in food is vegetables. If one looks at the chart (see Appendix 1), the high potassium foods are vegetables and fruits, with K/Na ratio highest for soy beans, banana, pumpkin, etc. All are very high. The poor potassium sources are animal or processed food, with K/Na ratio less than 1, including candies, cookies, canned goods, bread and bacon.

Why is food therapy popular? It is because it can increase the level of potassium in human cells, making it possible for cancer cells to revert to normal cells. Because this is a relatively new discovery, one will not find much information in scientific publications. On the other hand the sodium in the body is too high because of the many foods ingested which contain added salt, even including candies. Usually the salt is not noticed, but accumulates in the body. The potssium to sodium ratio for bread sold in the U.S. is 0.1 to 0.3, in other words, sodium is three to·ten times that of potassium. Apple pie also contains three times more sodium. Therefore the food in the potassium-poor section is not suited for sick people. Why am I emphasizing the ratio of potassium and sodium in food? Because it plays a role not only in cancer but also in high blood pressure, heart diseases, and diabetes, etc. In animal studies it was observed that when salt was added to food, the blood pressure rose, but when potassium was added, the blood pressure came down. It is not enough to reduce salt intake, one must also increase potassium intake. Eating more vegetables and fruits is a way to increase potassium intake.

Diabetes is due to insufficient secretion of insulin. The secretion of insulin is stimulated by potassium. Therefore deficient intake of potassium can be one of the causes of diabetes. In the U.S., the average intake of potassium over sodium is about 0.7, less than the body constitution, which is around 2.1. Cancer, heart diseases and diabetes are common in the U.S., and can be atributed to this factor in the diet. Chinese in general eat more rice, and vegetables. Their risk of getting these diseases is less.

(The above is a talk given at the Taiwan Sugar Company, Taipei in May, 1984.)

Chapter 9
Natural Food and the Health of Body and Mind

It is a common misconception that being human means that one must suffer the pains of birth, old age, illness and death. Actually, they are merely the price we pay for gratifying our appetites. If the natural way of eating is being followed, then not only aging and illnesses will no longer exist, but even the pains of birth and death can almost be reduced to zero.

The opening message may sound too simple to be true, yet it is what many doctors and scientists have discovered. This simple statement has also been verified by many scientific experiments. Our family of eight has followed the natural hygienic way of eating for over twenty years, and the experience is so rewarding that I am compelled to present our discovery here.

Natural food can be defined simply as all fresh vegetables, fruits, nuts, seeds and legumes that have not been subjected to heat nor processing. Cooked whole grain cereals such as brown rice and whole wheat flour are included in the category. But to really appreciate the value of natural food, it is necessary first to understand the nature of disease and physical deterioration. Therefore the next paragraph will review the causes and cures of diseases.

The orthodox medical profession after Pasteur has zealously upheld the theory that germs are the main cause of disease. As a result the physical condition of the patient is being overlooked. Medical research has been directed mainly toward the treatment of symptons. But after all these years of intensified research, only acute contagious diseases have been checked, while cases of chronic disorders are on the increase. This trend points out a serious defect in the prevailing approach. Increasingly, medical doctors and nutritionists are beginning to accept the fact that disease is the manifestation of the body's attempt to expel toxins. A condensed version of Dr. Bieler's opening message to the readers in "Food is Your Best Medicine" is given here: "As a practicing physician for over fifty years, I have reached three basic conclusions as to the cause and cure of disease. The first is that the primary cause of disease is not germs. Rather, disease is caused by a toxemia which results in cellular impairment and breakdown, thus paving the way for the multiplication and onslaught of germs. My second conclusion is that in almost all cases the use of drugs in treating patients is harmful. Drugs often cause serious side effects and sometimes even create new diseases. The dubious benefits they afford the patient are at best temporary. My third conclusion is that disease can be cured through the proper use of correct foods." Disease can be depicted as a friend in disguise; it is nature's warning. If, however, we continue to ignore this warning and eat the same old way, we are then doomed to self-destruction. Toxemia is caused by eating of cooked and processed food, especially of white sugar, polished rice and white flour. Natural foods are on the contrary not only nourishing, but also body cleansers. The roughly textured vegetable fibers are like brooms in cleaning the digestive tract. Fruits are rich in organic salts which can dissolve inorganic deposits and toxins. There is overwhelming evidence in favor of using natural food to treat disease. A Danish doctor cured herself of breast cancer with the use of a diet consisting entirely of raw vegetables, fruits and nuts.

Afterwards, she started a natural food sanitarium in Denmark. In another case, fresh carrot juice saved the life of a baby born with leukemia. Cases involving kidney and liver diseases, reumatism and asthma, to mention a few, are even more numerous. Even if one is not afflicted with any disease, one can benefit from natural foods in many ways. One will not only be freed from all diseases, but gain spirits of vitality and cheerfulness. Those who are "over the hill" can hope to feel and look ten to twenty years younger.

After we have exposed the real cause of disease, it is only natural to talk about disease-causing foods. They are traps on the road to health, or short paths to the grave.

REFINED SUGAR: Sugar is not only responsible for tooth-decay, but robs the body of vitamin B, disturbs calcium metabolism, and has a deleterious effect of the nervous system. Doctors have found that children who are allowed to have all the sweets they want become irritable and nervous. Once the sweets are removed, they are again well-behaved and poised. In the world of adults, nervousness, periodic depression, suspicion and even nervous breakdowns can be attributed to the eating of sugar. One of the most popular "myths" regarding sugar is the belief that it is an "energy food." Actually, white sugar is not a food, but a catalyst for burning what the body already has. Its effect on the body is very much like that of alcohol.

WHITE FLOUR & WHITE RICE: In the realm of nature, there is a balance between all constituents. Once the balance is broken, sickness occurs. Eating of white rice and white flour is one of the best examples of man's disruption of nature's balance. The nutrients necessary for the digestion of these food are being removed in the polishings, namely brans and germs. Without them, diseases, such as kidney and liver stones and arthritis make their appearance.

SALT: All the organic sodium chlorides the body needs can be found in raw vegetables. Salt not only slows down the digestion, but also increases the burden on the kidney. Varicose veins and hardening of arteries are the results of an excess intake of salt.

MILK: Milk is a factor in respiratory diseases, such as the common cold, asthma and tuberculosis. It is found to be the most mucous-forming food in the human diet. The source of trouble stems from the fact that cow's milk is vastly different from human mother's milk. As an example, it contains 300% more casein than does mother's milk. Although the calcium content of milk is high, its ratio to other minerals is out of proportion. Besides, in the process of pasteurization, the calcium is coverted to inorganic calcium which in turn is deposited in the joints. The best substitutes for human milk are goat's milk, carrot juice, seed milk, and fruit juices.

MEAT (all animal sources): Meat is the single most harmful food that is being shoveled down the human throat. Dr. Bernard in "Meat-eating is the Cause of Disease" stresses that meat-eating is responsible for cancer and diseases of the digestive tract, heart, liver and kidney. In the first place, the flesh of the dead animal still contains all the toxic waste of metabolism, especially uric acid. Our body absorbs most of the acid, and eventually when it crystalizes, it can cause intense pain. Also, we take in parasites that are originally in the animal. Secondly, putrefactive germs are often present (anywhere from one hundred thousand to ten million per gram). To make matters even worse, they are quite heat resistant. Thirdly, meat often comes for sick animals. Dr. Parrette in "Why I don't Eat Meat" disclosed that due to mass production, diseases are widely spreading among live stocks and chickens, specificly leukemia and cancerous tumors. Unfortunately, these disease are not only difficult to be detected in the early stages, but rather contagious when they appear. One cannot ignore the fact that cases of leukemia in children are on the increase.

Raw meat itself is bad enough, but most people eat it cooked. Whatever is left of its protein value is destroyed. Protein is essentially made up of more than twenty amino acids. Among these, there are eight ones which must be present at the same time in order to be used by the body. However, two of the eight happen to be heat-sensitive. Dr. Pottenger, using cats for experiments, found that cats on a cooked protein diet became sick and died prematurely. The diet included pasteurized milk, cheese, ice cream, eggs and meat.

In almost all cases, if meat is removed from the diet, one will experience improved health. As an example, a Hollywood movie star, after stopping eating meat, was surprised at the fact that her grapefruit-sized tumor of the womb had disappeared. During the second world war Denmark was forced on a non-meat diet for a year. During that time, the death rate dipped considerable; even the number of illnesses was lowered. When meat-eating was resumed during the second year, the death rate returned to the pre-war figure. Meat-eaters will sooner or later pay the price of health.

Meat-eating should not be tolerated in the first place for humanitarian reasons. Now even the pretext of eating for survival no longer stands, but there are enough evidences to prove that meat eating is actually a major cause of old age and disease. It is also economically disadvantageous. Indeed, in the process of feeding a cow, then slaughtering it for its meat, more than 70% of the feeds are wasted.

For those who have only known "civilized food," the above message may at first seem like a sentence of starvation. But if one looks around, one will find many nutritious and tasty "goodies." Everything from the vegetable kingdom will provide all that the body will ever need. Just for a start, I might mention a few. For protein-rich foods, bean sprouts, peanuts (must be raw), sesame seeds and sunflower seeds are excellent sources. Carrots, dandelions and all greens are good source of calcium. Perhaps I should use this opportunity to mention our daily menu, although it is offered only as a suggestion. For breakfast, we normally have a glass of fresh carrot juice and a piece of papaya, or any other seasonal fruit. Lunch consists mainly of two or three fruits, plus some dried fruits or sunflower seeds. Sometimes whole-wheat bread, carrot and celery sticks are added. Dinner is the biggest meal of the day. The main course is a big bowl of salad, made with anything from cucumbers, tomatoes and carrots to all sorts of greens. Then we have one or two dishes of lightly cooked vegetables. The dishes may seem almost tasteless to an outsider, but in time one finds them very delicious. Brown rice is a regular fare on the table, unless there are other starchy dishes. We often finish our meal with nuts and seeds.

This chapter is written only after reading numerous books and attending many lectures on the subject and after years of personal experience. However these few thousand words can serve the purpose of introducing the basic concepts behind natural food. As to the details of the diet, it is better to read some of the reference books.

Honolulu, Hawaii 1972

References:
1. Abrahamson, E.M., M.D. & Pezet, A.W.: Body, Mind and Sugar
2. Bernard, R.W., Ph.D.: Meat-Eating, A Cause of Disease
3. Bieler, H.G., M.D.: Food Is Your Best Medicine
4. Kirschner, H.E., M.D.: Live Food Juices
5. Kloss, J.: Back To Eden

6. Parrette, O.S., M.D.: Why I Don't Eat Meat
7. Richter, J.T., M.D.: Nature, The Healer
8. Shelton, H.M. M.D.: The Hygienic System
9. Walker, N.W., D.Sc.: Become Younger
10. Walker, N.W., D.Sc.: Diet and Salad Suggestions

Chapter 10
Raw Food - The Fountain of Youth

Americans are becoming more aware of their diet, and many are rebelling against the traditional style of eating. This was the cover story in the '72 December issue of Time magazine. The article went on to say the organic food movement has affected the American public in many ways. One indication of its influence is in the number of stores that specialize in health food, which increased from five hundred in 1965 to 3000 in 1972. At the same time, almost every major supermarket chain is either carrying or considering handling a line of health food items. As to the title, "The perils of eating, American style," the article is referring to the great percentage of Americans who are malnourished due to improper diet despite the wealth of America. It was pointed out that of 75 billion dollars in annual medical bills, 30 billion is the result of poor nutrition. Although doctors do not entirely agree on the precise role which diet plays in various diseases, it is accepted that diet is an important factor in heart disease, diabetes, tooth decay, and mental retardation.

The first example mentioned in the article was Paul Bragg. I will quote: "Paul Bragg, 91, claims that his lifeguard's physique was the result of two hours of daily exercise at Honolulu Waikiki Beach and his special diet. He eats natural food - fresh fruits, vegetables, seeds, but little meat and no salt; he plans to live to 120." I mention Dr. Bragg because I have attended his lectures on several occasions. He is a very humorous speaker. At his age, he still has loud and clear voice, and perfect vision. I remember him denouncing Americans' favorite diet: white sugar, white bread, coffee, soft drinks, hamburgers and hot dogs. Every year around Christmas, he leaves the country, because he cannot stand seeing people, especially kids, stuffing themselves with candies and other holiday "junk food." According to him, most people overeat. For example, he recommends only fruit juice or fruits for breakfast. He suggests that people would benefit from one day of fasting per week.

The search for everlasting youth has captured men's imagination from time immemorial. What the ancients could not find, modern scientists try to synthesize in the chemistry lab, or remake from nature in the operating room. In his search for the Fountain of Youth, man has overlooked one simple law of nature - you are what you eat! The seed of old age and decadence is sown right in the kitchen. The unsuspecting mother or housewife, while cooking the life out of food, unknowingly cook the youth, and life out of her family.

While it is true that cooked food can sustain life, it certainly serves less well to regenerate new cells - the most important factor in remaining youthful. Progressive degeneration of the cells and tissues results from diet consisting primarily of cooked food. Experiments have shown that sheep fed on cooked food died within five months. Of eight hogs that were experimented on, four that were on cooked food died of cholera within six months, while the other four on raw food were immune to the disease. Mice fed on white bread died sooner than mice that did not get any food at all. (The above information was taken from Dr. Carl Loeb's paper "How cooked food produces disease.") Wild animals eating all their food in their natural state are free from disease. Zoo animals fed on cooked food suffer from diseases similar to those that afflict modern man.

The miracle of raw food was often found accidentally. The discovery by a Swiss doctor, Dr. Bircher-Benner, more than 70 years ago is a classic. The incident happened to a dying patient with a chronic stomach disorder, who could not digest any food. A friend of the doctor suggested an ancient formula prescribed by the Greek philosopher Pythagoras more than 2000 years ago. Out of desperation he tried the formula - a mixture of mashed raw fruit, raw goat's milk and a little honey. Incredibly the food was digested and assimilated. The same food given before in cooked form passed undigested. This incident contradicted the general medical belief at that time - that cooked food is more digestible than raw food. Dr. Bircher-Benner being a man of science decided to do research in this area. Eventually he came up with the theory that green plants and fruits are the storehouse of the sun's energy. This energy is lost in fading, heating or fermentation. The Bircher-Benner Clinic of Zurich has been most successful in raw food therapy. (The International Congress of Nutritionists recently awarded him a gold medal for his contribution.)

With the advance of science, we know today that the intangible "something" in raw food is enzymes. Enzymes together with vitamins are the essential catalysts in digestion and assimilation of food. Enzymes are destroyed even at temperature slightly above 140° F (Water boils at 212° F). As an example, spinach and cabbage retain only 1/40 of their original food value after cooking. Because of raw food's high nutritional value, only a small amount is sufficient to supply bodily needs.

At this point, many readers may wonder aloud: "But where do I get my protein?" The misconception regarding protein is so deeply rooted, it would be worthwhile to mention the role of protein in a raw food diet. The generally accepted opinion on nutrition favors a diet of high protein intake, especially protein of animal origin. This belief is largely based on previous scientific research on animals. Unfortunately, in these experiments, the speed of growth was used as the sole criterion for judging the quality of protein, while the unfavorable effects of excess protein on a fully grown animal were not taken into account. (The above information was taken from "Eating Your Way to Health.") Based on new research, The Food and Nutrition Board of the International Research Council in Washington, D.C. has reduced the recommended protein consumption to nearly half of the original recommendation; the International Congress of Gerontologists has also requested the same. Even the scale of protein quality has been reversed; the green leaf and whole cereal proteins are rated higher than all animal sources of protein - meat, eggs, and milk. Research since 1967 at the Max Planck Institute for Nutritional Physiology has led to definite evidence that combinations of purely vegetable protein or mixtures of vegetable and other protein are consistenly higher in quality than all animal source of protein. The false sense of strength derived from meat-eating is an emergency reaction of the liver attempting to eliminate excess protein. Also meat contains toxic wastes of the animal, some of which is Xantin, closely related to the alkaloids in coffee and tobacco. Dr. Garten believes that we are imbibing narcotics when partaking in the eating of meat. It is thus expected that once meat is removed from the diet, the craving for tobacco and other stimulants will be gone.

Anatomically speaking, man is a fruit eater. This can be seen by the comparatively weak jaws, short canine teeth and clawless hands. Also the long intestine measuring twelve times the length of the spine as compared with only three times the length of th spine with meat-eaters. Meat-eating animals have short intestines which do not permit decomposition of food.

Once one forsakes the habit, he loses all desire for flesh food. Young children who have not lost their natural instinct have to be forced to eat meat. Dr. Bircher-Benner in "Diet for Children" stressed the fact that meat should never be given to children. It is especially harmful in the period of growth. It not only hurts them physically but mentally as well. Meat eating contributes a great deal to early maturity and accelerated aging. The Eskimos, living largely on meat and fat, age rapidly with an average life span of 27½ years. Many nomadic tribes living predominately on horse meat also mature early and die early. On the other hand people who live mostly on raw vegetables and fruits, and sparingly on meat enjoy a long and active life. As an example, the people in Hunza - situated in the midst of the Himalayas, eat most of their vegetables raw, due to scarcity of fuel. They also have plenty of fresh fruits and nuts. For them, meat is a rare luxury, available only once or twice a year, and only on special occasions. They not only look half their age, but enjoy an active life well into their hundreds. Who would believe that a man of 145 can still jump up to hit a volley ball?

Natural food is the best answer to shortage of food and high medical cost. Even if one cannot go on a complete natural food diet, one can still benefit greatly. Ultimately, fruits, nuts and raw vegetables should comprise the major portion of the diet. However, it takes some time initially to adjust to raw food; therefore one must go through a transition period (approximately two years). The following are some simple rules to ease the change-over:

1. Increase the amount of fresh vegetables and fruits steadily until they comprise at least 50% of the diet.

2. Steam cooking is the best, the Chinese way of quick frying comes next.

3. Avoid drinking liquids with the meal, as this dilutes the digestive juices.

4. Eat only when hungry, allowing at least 5 hours between meals.

5. Eat fruits before the main meal, as fruits take much less time to digest.

6. Eat not more than three servings of meat per week. According to Dr. Bragg, this is the maximum amount the human body can tolerate.

The following are some suggestions for the three meals: Breakfast: This is the most important meal of the day in the sense that it can control the whole day's mood and spirit. Fruits are the most ideal, perhaps with the addition of some seeds and grain porridge. Lunch: The main dish could be a fruit or vegetable salad, supplemented with dried fruits, nuts, or some whole-grain cereal. Dinner: The menu could be like lunch, with one or two dishes of steamed or lightly cooked vegetables added.

Once one has started on the diet, one can expect many changes, including easier digestion, good appetite, sound sleep, free bowel movement, natural glossy hair, improved dental health and sparkling eyes. Mentally, there is a general cheerfulness, alertness and well-being. Initially one can also expect weight loss, but unless one was overwight to begin with, the loss is temporary. There will also be times when one will not feel his best; this symptom indicates that a substantial amount of poison is being eliminated from the body. This will pass quickly and one gains greater energy.

Mother nature is fair and just. Health and happiness are yours when you follow her laws. Disease and sorrow set in when the laws are broken. The choice is yours.

Honolulu, Hawaii 1973

Chapter 11
Vegetarian Food Is Your Best Medicine

"Vegetarian food is good medicine" can be discussed from the perspective of individual health and planetary health. (It is undeniable that our survival depends on planetary health.)

Vegetarian Food and Individual Health

We begin by looking at individual health. The concept that "food is better than medicine" is present both in the East and the West. That food can affect our health is not a new concept. Why can vegetarian food keep us in health? In Chinese villages, there is a saying: "Vegetables and tofu will keep you in peace." For thousands of years, Chinese peasants ate a simple diet of rice and vegetables, with the exception of special celebrations, and thus were mostly vegetarians. Unless there were famines or epidemics, most people were in good health.

When an agricultural society becomes an industrial society, not only lifestyle changes, but food habits also change drastically. In the past, meat and fish were available only during special ocassions; now they are eaten everyday. White sugar used to be a luxury food; now it can be bought anytime. Brown rice and whole wheat are replaced with white rice and white flour. In a short twenty to thirty years, these diet changes have

71

affected health conditions in general. Heart diseases, diabetes, cancer, excess weight, and premature aging are now common. On the surface life expectancy has increased, but it is due to a lowered infant mortality rate. At least in the U.S., the life expectancy for those over forty has not increased in the last fifty years. It is doubtful that progress in science and medicine has actually increased life expectancy.

It has now been proven that proper vegetarian food can not only prevent disease but can also cure disease. Books and articles published in this area are too numerous to mention. One will find these books in any bookstores in the U.S. There might be differences among nutritionists on specifics. For example, some insist on raw food, where others insist on cooked food. Still others emphasize brown rice, or wheatgrass. But all of them provide evidence that vegetarian food can treat diseases.

Let us use the example of a book written by Henry Bieler, M.D.. In "Food is Your Best Medicine" Dr. Bieler wrote: "Allopathic medicine invariably has side effects. Food, on the other hand does not have this problem." In his fifty years as a practicing physician, he has used food to help people with various illnesses. His patients included Hollywood stars, such as Gloria Swanson, who has been his devoted student since 1927. She not only lived a long time but also stayed young. In the book, vegetables were used as medicine. One chapter is titled: Vegetables As Do-it-Yourself Therapy. There were many examples of using vegetables to treat sickness. He used fresh alfalfa (it was difficult to obtain fresh greens in late fall), fresh milk and whole wheat bread to cure a farmer's gangrene of long standing. After that, the farmer stayed away from pork, white sugar, and white flour.

Dr. Bieler's way of treating diabetes was to let the patient rest for two or three days, taking only broth made from celery, parsley, green beans, and zucchini. The patient then returned to a normal diet based on vegetables. When urine sugar level rose, the person was to return to the vegetable broth diet for two or three days. Through this trial and error, a diet was found that keeps the blood sugar level normal. His theory is that the main constituent of the pancreas is potassium. Only when its function is below normal, one has diabetes. Increased potassium intake can stimulate the pancreas to return to normal function. Vegetables and fruits are the richest sources of potassium, containing hundreds of times that of meat and fish. Dr. Bieler reported a case of a Hollywood movie star dissolving a uterus tumor the size of grapefruit by going on a vegetarian diet.

Dr. Bieler himself was a vegetarian. When the book came out in 1965, he was already approaching eighty years of age. He only died recently. His recommendaton for food is to eat more fresh vegetables and whole grains, and to avoid refined foods and meat.

There are mainly two schools of thought on using vegetarian food as medicine. One theory espouses eating only raw food, particularly sprouts. Of course there are many successful cases. This way of eating may not suit the Chinese taste. The other theory uses mainly brown rice, millet, buckwheat, and cooked vegetables. It is known as a Macrobiotic diet. Food choices are recommended to tailor to the environment, and the season. The variety of food includes seeds (sesame, etc.), sea vegetables, vegetables and roots (carrots, etc.), dried fruits, fresh fruits, grains, and beans. Oil and salt are used sparingly in cooking, with boiling or steaming considered the best. Miso is used for seasoning. The macrobiotic way of eating is widely known in the U.S.; most cities have a macrobiotic food center. Many cancer patients have found recovery through this diet.

To understand further the role of vegetarian food in preventing and treating illnesses, one must consider potassium and sodium. It has been mentioned already that plants contain the highest levels of potassium. Using the ratio of potassium to sodium as an indicator, pumpkin is 360, soy bean 331, banana 380, orange, 221. On the contrary the ratios for meat, chicken and fish never exceed three to five. Ham is 0.3, lobster 0.9. The above information was taken from the U.S. Deparment of Agriculture. In summary, most of the fruits and vegetables have a potassium to sodium ratio of over 200. Refined and processed food such as cookies and cakes and canned goods have ratios less than 1. There are not too many discussions of potassium and sodium ratios in the scientific journals, as yet. It is a relatively new field of study.

Why does potassium play an important role in our health? For cells to perform normally, they need to concentrate potassium and expel sodium. In the cells, potassium to sodium ratio is about 10 times. When cell membranes are damaged, potassium is leaked and the cells start to divide. Dividing cells and cancer cells have a lower ratio of potassium to sodium compared to normal cells. Intracellular potassium-sodium ratio can control cell growth. That cancer cells grow in an uncontrolled manner is probably related to the lowered potassium-sodium ratio. There are now epidemiological data indicating there is an inverse correlation between potassium intake and incidence of cancer. Potassium may have a protective effective towards cancer. That vegetables are used in the treatment of cancer is related to the high potassium content. Generally high blood pressure is related to high intake of sodium, while potassium can reduce blood pressure. People on a vegetarian diet usually do not have blood pressure problems, if salt is not over used. According to studies in the U.S., potassium intake should be higher than sodium by at least 2 times. However the actual intake is 0.7. It is no wonder that heart diseases is the number one cause of death in the U.S.

Vegetarian diet and the health of the planet

The above is a brief discussion of why a vegetarian diet is related to individual health. Next we will look at the relation between a vegetarian diet and planetary health.

We are more and more aware that the earth has limited resources, expecially fossil fuel, fertile soil and clean water. We also know that there are many people who do not have enough to eat. Is this due to lack of food or poor distribution? Frances Moore Lappe in "Diet for a Small Planet" pinpointed the problem: the issue is not lack of food but a waste of the planet's resources. Using grains to feed cattle, sheep, and hogs is very wasteful. On the average it takes seven pounds of grains to get one pound of meat. Beef is even more wasteful. One pound of beef requires 16 pounds of soy beans. Fifty percent of agricultural products in the U.S. are used for feeding livestock.

In order to increase crop yields, large quantities of chemical fertilizers and pesticides are used. This not only pollutes the soil, but also uses fossil fuel (Chemical fertilizers and pesticides are by-products of fossil fuel). At the same time, poisoned fertile soil cannot regenerate. Every year much topsoil is lost. As production decreases every year, more and more chemical fertilizers are used, causing a vicious cycle.

Water is another precious resource. Water for drinking and farming becomes scarcer every year. The underground water level in some parts of the U.S. is lowered six inches to six feet every year. The production of meat uses a lot of water. One pound of beef takes 2500 gallons of water, and one pound of soy bean takes only 1/10 to ⅓ of that. Fifty percent of water consumption in the U.S. is used for meat production. Experts are warning of not enough water. In this situation, we must re-examine our food habits.

Plant food requires far less of the earth's resources to produce than animal food. Here is another example: to produce one calorie of protein from soy bean takes two calories, from other beans or grains 3.5 calories, from pork 35 calories, and beef 78 calories.

In the past, it was often thought that animal sources of protein are higher than plant sources of protein. This is a half truth. Protein is formed from amino acids, eight of which must be present, called essential amino acids. Grains and beans all contain very high levels of protein, but not balanced in amino acid distribution. Legumes have higher levels of lysine and lower levels of sulfur containing amino acids. Grains are the opposite. If eaten alone, their protein value is diminished. If eaten together, the protein values are increased tremendously. Usually one would not eat only beans and not grains, or vice versa. Therefore the value of plant protein is not less than meat.

All the traditional foods of the world are balanced in this way. In China tofu and rice are eaten, in Mexico, corn tortillas and beans, in the Middle East, tahini or garbanzo beans with bread, and in India dal and rice or chappati. As long as one is not eating an extreme diet, plant food can provide all that the body needs, including protein. According to one report, Americans usually consume more than twice as much protein as the body needs. Even if all meats are removed from the diet without any other changes, the intake of protein is still more than what the body needs. Excess protein not only wastes energy, but also harms the body, especially the kidneys.

Our dietary habits on a small scale affect our health, while on the large scale, the health of our life support system, the earth. We should give it serious thought. Furthermore from the Buddist point of view, eating without killing is connected with liberation. Regardless, a vegetarian diet is the solution to all of these problems. A vegetarian diet is the best medicine for life.

Chapter 12
"Let Your Body Be Your Own Doctor" - The Story of Dr. Ann Wigmore

"Dear Dr. Ann,

Let me introduce myself. Wheatgrass has made me into a new man. Eleven months ago, I had diabetes, my circulation was so bad, I was afraid I was going to lose a leg. At that time I spent sixty to seventy dollars every month on medication and vitamins, but my health continued to worsen . . . ." This letter of gratitude was written by a man from New Orleans, Louisiana. After following the wheatgrass and raw food diet prescribed by Dr. Ann Wigmore, his blood sugar returned to normal.

There are many such "Dear Dr. Ann" letters from around the world. These people, after practicing the simple and inexpensive way of eating fresh food, regained their health. Who is this Dr. Ann? Located in the midst of the old cultural city of Boston is a five story, nineteenth century building. On a cold wintery day, if you step through the door, you will find yourself in a green world surrounded with catus plants and trays of green sprouts and wheatgrass. The air is filled with the sweet smell of grass. This is the Hippocrates Health Institute established by Dr. Ann Wimore more than twenty years ago. Every year approximately one thousand people come to regain their health. Their illnesses include diabetes, low blood sugar, asthma, allergy, constipation, headaches, high blood pressure, low blood pressure, arthritis, heart diseases, all kinds of ulcers, gall stones, kidney infections, epilepsy, and cancer. Almost 100% of them gain some relief. H.H.I. follows the philosophy of "Let Food Be Thy Medicine," uttered 2500 years ago by Hippocrates. Dr. Ann's own introduction is as follows: "Our basic approach to healing is following that of Hippocrates. If the body is provided with proper tools, fresh, uncooked and unrefined foods, the body is its own best doctor."

H.H.I. is a non-profit, educational and research institution, focused on finding the most healthful, economical, and nutritious foods. Consequently, it has eliminated meat and all refined food. It has also completely adopted the use of fresh fruits and vegetables. Its educational policy is pursued along four directions: 1. residential - guest basis; 2. residential - student basis; 3. residential - working-staff basis; 4. education through correspondence. People who come to H.H.I. rely on fresh and nutritious food, in particular sprouts grown indoors, which are rich in enzymes, vitamins, minerals, but low in starch, fat and protein. Residential guests or students after three weeks of learning in residence, can continue at home. They can move into staff positions also, but not for more than six months duration.

The nutritious organic food includes buckwheat sprouts, sunflower seed sprouts, and wheatgrass. The above are all planted in trays of soil and harvested after one week to ten days. The other sprouts are mung beans, lentil, alfalfa, fenugreek, garbanzo, and adzuki beans. Besides these, there are fruits, sesame and sunflower seeds. Rejuvelac, made with wheat and full of enzymes, is the main beverage. To make rejuvelac, one soaks one cup of wheat berries with three cups of water for 24 hrs at room temperature, best at 75° F. The resulting water is full of vitamin C and enzymes. The same wheat can be soaked for two more times, 24hrs each time. One can also sprout the wheat first before soaking. To sprout, cover the wheat with water overnight. Drain excess water and cover for two days. The sprouted wheat can be used as cereal or to make rejuvelac. The ratio of water to sprouted wheat is 2 to 1. All the foods served at H.H.I. are not cooked. Three years ago they removed the stove.

Dr. Ann's own personal story began during World War I in East Europe. She was born very frail. Her parents, thinking that she was not going to live long, left her in the care of her grandma and immigrated to the U.S. Under the loving care of grandma, she lived. In her eyes, her grandmother was the greatest physician. She knew the use of medicinal plants, being the doctor in the village. After she grew up, there was a period of two years during which her home became a battleground between the Germans and the Russians. During that dark period, she and her grandma lived on tree bark and grass. That experience of living on greens left an unforgetable impression. As a teenager, she came to the U.S. to join her parents. After one year of living on modern food - Coca Cola, donuts and other refined foods, her health deteriorated. She also lost four teeth. She started to pray to God for help. Several years later after she moved to Boston, she read a passage in the Bible where King Nebuchadnezar, after following the advice of a voice from heaven to eat grass, recovered from his illnesses. She had the realization that if grass cured the King's sickness, it could also work on others. She began to collect grass seeds and found wheatgrass to grow the fastest. The roots are strong and the leaves rich in chlorophyll. Her personal health also benefited from experimentation with wheatgrass juice. She had more energy and could work more hours. She went on to receive further training, earned a degree in Naturopathy, and a degree in divinity.

That chlorophyll from wheatgrass juice has curative power has been demonstrated in many research institutions. Dr. G.H. Earp Thomas is a soil scientist. He analyzed over 100 constitutents of wheatgrass, which is rich in protein and enzymes. Wheatgrass is a complete food. The structure of chlorophyll is very similar to that of haemoglobin. Dr. Frans Miller found that the ability of chlorophyll to reverse anemia in animal studies is similar to that of iron.

At H.H.I., wheatgrass juice is used both orally and as implants. To take orally, dilute one tablespoon of wheatgrass juice with half cup of rejuvelac. After two days increase to ¼ cup juice to ¾ cup water. To take as implant: Take first a water enema to cleanse the colon. Take in ½ to one cup of wheatgrass juice, retain in the colon for 20 to 30 minutes. People with serious illnesses can take another implant after two hours. Jack Chambers from Canada visitied H.H.I. in December of 1974. He was suffering from Maelosytic Leukemia. The cancer was discovered in 1973 Spring, and he had received chemotherapy and Laetrile, but only with partial success. While staying at H.H.I., he lived on raw foods, and took wheatgrass implants four times a day. He felt better after only a few days. Five weeks later his blood test at Boston's Brusch Clinic showed there was no more cancer. Two months before arriving in Boston his blood test still showed cancer cells in the blood.

Why the use of wheatgrass as medicine and fresh vegetables, fruits, and sprouts as food? Sprouts are one of the most nutritious and economical foods. For example, Dr. Bruck from Yale University found vitamin B increased 100% after sprouting. Just think, one pound of seeds produces seven pounds of food.

To Sprout: Use a wide-mouthed jar, the size depends on one's need. Cover the jar with cheese cloth or mesh. Place a few spoonfuls of seeds in the jar. Smaller seeds such as alfalfa, radish and celery need to be soaked for only four hours. Beans such as adzuki beans, mung beans, soy beans, and lentil, as well as peas and wheat need to be soaked for ten hours. After soaking, rinse twice a day. The sprouts are ready for eating after one week. Place in indirect sunlight before serving to increase the level of chlorophyll.

Methods to plant wheatgrass and green sprouts: Use a tray about one inch in height, filled with fertile soil, preferably soil from the forest, not treated with chemical fertilizer. Chemical fertilizers are normally somewhat water soluble, easily absorbed into the soil upsetting the natural balance. Chemical fertilizers also produce acid residues, making the soil unsuitable for the growth of earthworms and micro-organisms. Earthworms and micro-organisms are important for the health of the soil. To enrich the soil, one can add leaves or green manure and alternate planting. Place soaked seeds, such as sunflower, buckwheat, or wheat, on moistened soil, covering it with ten layers of wet newspaper and plastic sheet. After three days, remove the paper, and place near the window. Water once or twice a day and harvest the green sprouts after one to two weeks. The used soil can be stored in a plastic container and re-used after three weeks. The soil gets richer after each planting, because the roots are left in the soil as fertilizer.

The success stories of Dr. Ann are too numerous to mention. Two more examples will be given here: Mrs. Audrey from Massachusetts had suffered from serious asthma for many years. Sometimes she needed to be taken to the hospital and placed under an oxygen mask. In the three weeks that she came to H.H.I., she did not have asthma and it never recurred again. This was three years ago.

Mrs. Gavin first discovered that she had cancer of the uterus in December, 1970. Her doctor recommended surgery. She postposed the date to one month later, hoping to find alternatives. She started changing her diet, and came to H.H.I. and told her doctor to change the date to June. The doctor replied that she might not be alive by then. After three weeks at H.H.I. she went back to her doctor for another checkup. The doctor was unhappy. He emphasized that if she did not follow his advice, she should change doctors. However, the results of that test showed the uterus to be normal, with no sign of cancer.

The nutrition system followed at H.H.I. does not include meat. Why? The following are some explanations.

Meat is the most wasteful and unclean food.

Meat is the corpse of dead animals. It contains not only millions of putrifactive bacteria, but also biological waste products and parasites. For example, trichinosis is entirely a meat-eaters' disease. At least 60% of Americans have these parasites in their muscles. The young larve of trichinea enter through ingestion of meat, then penetrate the intestinal wall, carried by the blood stream and reside in different parts of the body. The unpleasant symptons are fever, muscle pain and swelling. Meat (including those of the sea animals) contain concentrated levels of pesticide, herbicide and other chemical pollutant. A recent issue of Time magazine reported on the residents of Mitsumata after eating mercury-containing fish. Over ten years, hundreds have died, while others are blinded, deaf, mute or insane. Only recently it was found that a chemcal factory had been discharging waste water containing methyl mercury. This factory has paid over six billion U.S. dollars in damages, and will soon close its doors.

Meat decomposes in the intestine; the resulting waste matter then gets into the blood stream. Dr. Moore of the Harvard University Laboratory of Physiology discovered that after ingestion of meat, the human heart beat increased 25 to 50%. This lasted 15 to 20 hours. His explanation: "This phenomenon (of rapid heart beat) indicates poison in the body." This is further evidence that meat is toxic.

From the environmental and economic perspective, to support a meat eater requires six times more land than supporting a vegetarian. Imagine, to produce one pound of beef requires 20 pounds of grain. If the resources of the earth were equitably distributed, there would be enough food for everyone. At this time when the world has serious food shortages in dfferent parts of the world, how can one eat meat for humanitarian reasons? On the contrary, one pound of seed can produce seven pounds of food. Just the numbers should convince thinking people to stop eating meat, let alone the health and humanitarian reasons.

Why eat raw foods? Fresh foods are rich in enzymes. Enzymes help to breakdown larger molecules, such as starch and fat. Enzymes become inactive with heat, above 60° C or 140° F. Dr. Ann in "Be Your Own Doctor" emphasizes that cooked foods lack enzymes, and therefore cannot be fully digested. The residues remain in the intestine to rot. Eating only cooked food over long periods can cause all kinds of tumor growth. She has seen cancer cells grow in cooked food but not in the corresponding raw food. The cooking process also reduces the utilization of protein. Protein is made up of 20 amino acids, eight of which are essential; they must be present together to form protein. Of these, two are heat sensitive.

In Dr. Ann's dictionary, there is no such word as "incurable." Cancer for example, is rapidly becoming the number one cause of death in the U.S., overtaking heart diseases. The normal procedure is surgery (Edward Kennedy's son lost one leg due to surgery) or removal of the cancerous growth from the breast, uterus, etc. It may be treated with radiation or poisonous chemotherapy. The treatments used for cancer often are more frightening than the disease itself. Even if one is saved from cancer, one is crippled or disfigured from the treatment. Even more of concern is that if the body chemistry is not changed, the cancer can return.

The "miracles" that take place everyday at H.H.I. provide hope for those suffering from cancer or other "incurables." Just like other diseases, cancer can also be treated by natural methods. At H.H.I., 50 to 60% of the resident guests have advanced cancer. They come after trying everything else. If they can follow the raw food diet and wheatgrass juice treatment, they can regain their health. According to Dr. Ann, even in the serious stages of cancer, it takes only about one year to recover. Those with early stages can recover in a matter of weeks. Maya, one of the staff at H.H.I, had cancer one year ago. Her right ovary had been removed at age fifteen due to cancer. Sixteen years later, her uterus and the area of the right ovary developed cancer. She had been in and out of hospitals many times because she had other complications, including loss of kidney function such that water is retained, a swollen abdomen, low blood sugar and arthritis. After all her money was spent, she turned to natural medicine. She started eating natural food, raw sprouts, and drinking sprout juices. One year ago she came to H.H.I. to work as a volunteer, and to regain her health. She lookes like a new person, looking only in her twenties for a thirty-two year old. Because of her own experience of suffering, she is dedicating her life to helping others.

Dr. Ann Wigmore is not the only one who has had success in using nature's green grass and vegetables for healing. Dr. H.E. Kirschner, M.D. in "Nature's Healing Grasses" shares his experience of using green grass in treating all kinds of illnesses. The greens are taken in the form of green drink, made with weeds such as dandelion, comfrey, nettle, alfalfa, watercress, parsley, spinach, and lambs quarter. These greens are blenderized with pineapple juice (for flavoring only). Dr. Max Gerson,

M.D. in "A Cancer Therapy" describes in detail another approach to treating cancer. Using fresh vegetable juices, and fruit juices, he has reversed many terminal cancer cases.

Cambridge, Massachusetts, 1976

Chapter 13
The Effect of Cookware and Cooking Fuel on Food

In the cooking process, one needs to be concerned about the effect of cookware and cooking fuel on the energy of food. Most people are not aware of the importance of cookware, although some may be aware of the hazards of aluminum cookware because of its toxicity.

Dr. Rudolf Hauschka in "Nutrition" compares the biological effect of water boiled in different cookware and using different cooking fuel. To test the effects of fuel on living systems, water was boiled in glassware for twenty minutes with different fuels. The water was then cooled to room temperature and used to water wheat seeds. The growth of wheat seedlings and roots was measured after ten days. The fuels used in the experiment were electricity, gas, coal, wood and straw. The control group was watered with unheated water. The results are as follows: wheatgrass grew the least with electrically boiled water, even less than unheated water. Gas flame-cooked water produced the next shortest sprouts, but similar to the control. Coal-cooked water produced slightly taller sprouts than gas flame-cooked water. Straw flame-cooked water produced the tallest sprouts, taller than wood flame-cooked water. From this we can see that of the commonly used fuels, electric heat is most damaging to food. The traditional wood fire produced better growth of wheatgrass. The Macrobiotic school of thought emphasizes that sick people should avoid electric heat for cooking. Now it is clear why.

Another experiment studies the influence of cookware on the growth of wheatgrass. The results are as follows: gold is the best. The good news is that gold-plated spoons used for stiring food have a beneficial effect. Wooden spoons have similar effect. It is no wonder emperors of the past used goldware for eating. That was not only an enjoyment, but also consistent with nutritional science. From the result of the growth of wheatgrass, the cookware second to gold is clay pottery, followed by ceramic, enamel, glass, copper, iron, stainless steel; the worst is aluminum. Water boiled in aluminum pots inhibited the growth of wheatgrass.

That water boiled in aluminum pots produced the poorest growth is understandable. Aluminum is made from clay at extremely high temperature. On the surface it is a metal, but quickly forms clay, and therefore is not very stable. Most people have had the experience of watching potato and barley cooked in aluminium pots turn black. Spinach or tomato can dissolve the surface of the pot, leaving pock marks in the pot. There was a report of people getting food poisoning from eating food stored in aluminum pots. Clay pots are closest to nature. The boiled water in clay pots is second only to gold pots.

Dr. Hauschka also made recommendations regarding the harvest and cooking of vegetables. Flowers and leaves such as cauliflower, broccoli, and greens are best eaten raw. At most, they should be quickly stir-fried or lightly steamed for a few minutes. They are best harvested in the morning, the nutrient content being highest. Root vegetables such as carrots are best stir-fried or steamed; cooking time is slightly longer, about ten minutes. It is best to harvest in the afternoon.

This study did not mention the Microwave oven and its effect on food. I did an experiment on my own, comparing water cooked in a Microwave oven and over electric heat and its effect on the growth of wheatgrass. The containers were all glass, cooking over electric heat for twenty minutes and by microwave for ten minutes. The results of the wheatgrass growth are as follows: In ten days, the Microwaved-water produced wheatgrass only 60% in height and 50% in weight compared to the electrically-cooked water. This experiment was repeated with the same result. The microwave oven is the newest product of technology, even further from nature. It no surprise that it is most damaging to life.

Houston, 1987

Quick, Throw the Aluminium Pot Away

In 1989, while travelling and living in India, I personally experienced aluminium poisoning. It made me more concerned about this problem, and made me more alert when visiting. I always check to see if there are aluminium utensils in the kitchen. When encountering people who have undiagnosed sickness, I always ask if they use aluminium cookware.

What are the symptoms of aluminium poisoning? The initial reaction is that of gas, upset stomach, constipation and tiredness. If continued, one will notice backache, pressure in the chest and depression. Over long term exposure, it can lead to Alzeheimer's disease. It is difficult to detect aluminium poisoning, because it shows up differently in different people. It will show up first in the weakest link, such as liver, spleen, pancreas, kidneys, heart, etc. It will also damage the nervous system. In my own experience of ingesting aluminium after two to three weeks, my hives that had not bothered me for twenty years flared up, itching all over the body and causing swollen eyes and lips. As mentioned, depression is another symptom of poisoning. I met a German woman who after living in India and Nepal for one year, became suicidal. Doctors could not trace the cause. After suggesting it could be due to aluminium poisoning, she understood. She took herbal medicine for elimination of aluminium and had good results.

Use of aluminium cookware in heating water, rice and vegetables is not the only source of poisoning. Drinking aluminium canned beverages can also expose one to it. Usually, the symptoms are reduced within about two months after stopping intake of aluminum. Taking vitamin C can speed up the elimination.

There was a professor who always exhibited two bowls of goldfish during his lecture on aluminium. One bowl was filled with water boiled in glass and the other in aluminium. After one hour one of the goldfish was dead. Can you guess which one?

Denver, July 1991

Chapter 14
Recipes

To put eating healthy food in practice, one must first gather the necessary ingredients. The basic ingredients are grains, legumes, seeds, nuts, sea vegetables, soy bean products, fresh vegetables, fruits, sprouts and seasoning such as miso. Legumes are best eaten after sprouting, easier to digest and more nutritious. To cook legumes, soak them overnight, pour off the water next day, and keep it at room temperature for one day. In the sprouting process, protein molecules are broken down into amino acids, and are thus easier to digest. Vitamin content also increases. Miso not only seasons but helps to eliminate radioactive materials from the body. Sea vegetables contain rich sources of mineral, and supplement whatever may be missing in land-produced food.

GRAINS: rolled oats, millet, buckwheat, barley, rye, wheat, brown rice, corn, etc.

LEGUMES: adzuki beans, mung beans, lentil, black beans, peas, and chick peas.

SEEDS AND NUTS; sesame seeds, sunflower seeds, pumpkin seeds, almond, pine nuts, cashew nuts, walnuts, and peanuts.

SPROUTING:

There are two methods of sprouting. The first is easiest, using water only with no requirement for soil. The following can be sprouted this way: lentil, fenugreek, mung bean, and alfalfa. One need only a wide-mouthed glass jar, four to ten cups in volume. Take a piece of cheese cloth or nylon stocking and secure with a rubber band at the top. Wash the seeds then soak in water overnight. Alfalfa seeds need to be soaked only for five hours. Use ½ to one cup of seeds, except alfalfa (¼ cup is sufficient). Remove the water after soaking, and rince once or twice a day. After one week the sprouts are ready for eating. Some seeds require even less time than one week, just three to four days. The vitamin contents are highest in young sprouts. It also has pain relieving properties. In harvesting, rinse off the skins and store in plastic containers in the refrigerator.

The second method of sprouting requires soil. Although it may take a little extra work, the green sprouts of sunflower seeds and buckwheat sprouts are delicious, worthy of the extra work. Wheatgrass is also grown this way. Tools needed are trays made of iron, plastic, wood, or paper wrapped with plastic sheets. The size does not matter. For an average family, if one plants three days per week, one 18-inch square tray per planting is sufficient. Place one inch of soil on the tray, and moisten with water. The seeds can be one to two cups, soaked overnight first, then spread evenly over the moistened soil. Cover them with wet newspapers and a plastic sheet. In the winter, place in the room; in the summer, place it outside. Remove the sheets after three or four days and place in indirect sun. Harvest after seven to ten days, cut above the roots and rinse well. The used soil can be placed in a bin for three months and used again.

SUGGESTIONS FOR BREAKFAST:

Breakfast is usually simple. In the spring and summer months, some fruits and muesli are sufficient. In the fall and winter one can have five-grain porridge. Energy soup can be served in any season. In the cold season, make it with warm liquid to have warm soup.

1. FIVE-GRAIN PORRIDGE: Choose five types of grains, and then grind coarsely in the blender. Cook with sufficient water to make porridge. This can be sweetened with raisins or molasses, or made salty with miso and sesame oil. One can also add ground sesame or pumpkin seeds.

2. MUESLI: This recipe was developed by the famous Swiss nutritionist Dr. Bircher-Benner. It can be eaten by adults and children, even three meals a day by those who are sick. One adult serving: two tablespoons of oats soaked in four tablespoons of water overnight. The next morning add one Tbsp. of seeds or nuts, half a lemon, one fruit, grated (banana, apple, papaya, or any seasonal fruit). Sweeten with honey if desired.

3. SPROUTED WHEAT WITH RAISINS: This is served cooked or uncooked. Soak wheat in water overnight. Pour off the water the next day, and cover for two days without additional watering. The sprouts are ready for eating.

4. ENERGY SOUP: Use fruits such as apples, pears, watermelon or fruit juices as a base. Place in the blender and add greens, sprouts, and a little seaweeds, and half an avocado. Blenderize quickly and serve fresh.

SUGGESTIONS FOR LUNCH AND DINNER

If possible, make lunch the main meal, and eat a light dinner.

1. Nori-wrapped rice balls, vegetable salad, avocado seasoned with miso-peanut sauce.

2. Miso-seaweed-tofu soup, five-grain rice, mixed vegetable delight, carrot sticks.

3. Energy soup: Mix one Tbsp. of miso in one cup of hot water. Place in blender and add sprouts, vegetables, sunflower

seeds or sesame seeds and little seaweed to blenderize. This is the salty version of energy soup. For the sweet version, use watermelon or other fruits as base, the rest is the same. Energy soup was created by Dr. Ann Wigmore; it contains rich nutrients and is easily digested. One can also flavor with ginger, basil or other herbs. For colder days, making it with warm liquid is more comfortable.

SEASONING:

MISO PEANUT (or sesame) SAUCE or dressing: Mix two Tbsp. of miso with four Tbsp. of peanut or sesame butter, one tsp. of minced ginger and half a cup of water. Mix well. For salad dressing, thin with more water. This sauce can be used on noodles, or poured over steamed vegetables (cauliflower, pumpkin, broccali, etc.).

SALAD DRESSING: Here are a few recipes for dressings.

Sesame and sunflower seed dressing: Soak half a cup of sesame seeds and half a cup of sunflower seeds in water for five hours. Drain and cover for five hours, let the seeds sprout a little. Blenderize with one cup of water and place at room temperature for eight hours. Let it ferment slightly and season.

Potato dressing: Remove the skin from cooked potato and mash. Add olive oil sesame, cashew, lemon juice, brown sugar and dulse for seasoning.

Cucumber dressing: Pat cucumber then add a little salt. Mix in seaweed, sesame oil, brown sugar, and vinegar; blenderize quickly.

ADDITIONAL RECIPES:

Sweet Jewel Soup: half cup each of lotus seeds, white fungus, adzuki beans, peanuts, chestnuts and dried lily bulb. Boil with six cups of water. Depending on one's preference, one can increase or decrease water and sweeten with molasses or brown sugar.

Sweet Jewel Porridge: Same ingredients as above, except add half a cup of sweet rice.

Pumpkin Soup: Cook cubed pumpkins in water. Add fresh peas and miso peanut sauce to taste.

Bean Soup: Cube carrots. Use lentil or peas, soaked overnight and sprouted slightly. Heat a little butter in pan, add curry powder and carrot cubes, then add beans and water. Cook until done. One can add black mushroom, dried lily flowers and seasonings such as miso or soy sauce.

WHEAT SPROUTS AND THEIR USE:

1. Wheat sprout milk: Blenderize one cup of water with one cup of wheat sprouts. Filter out the pulp and sweeten with dates or molasses.

2. Wheat sprout suncake: Blenderize sprouted wheat with water (2 cups sprouted wheat with ½ cup water). Shape into a cookie about the width of a rice bowl. Dried under sun or in slow oven.

3. Sprouted wheat bread: When making bread, add sprouted wheat, whole or ground.

4. Sprouted wheat balls: Blenderize wheat sprouts (two cups of sprouted wheat and ½ cup of water); add one cup of ground sunflower seeds or sesame seeds. Add bread crumbs if desired. Form into one-inch balls and bake in slow oven, about 300° F for fifteen minutes.

5. Vegetarian balls: Grind sprouted wheat. Add an equal amount of ground walnuts or sunflower seeds. Season with ginger, or basil and miso, or sesame oil. The balls made from the mixture can be fried or baked. If minced Chinese cabbage and bean threads are added, one can make dumplings or wontons.

Chapter 15
Food As Medicine

LEMON: Lemon has many uses in health; One can add a few drops of lemon juice to drinking water. Used externally, lemon juice can draw out pus from boils, pimples, and skin allergies. Used internally, lemon juice can treat constipation, ulcer, fever. To take, add juice of one lemon in one glass of warm water. Sweeten with honey or molasses. For sore throat, one can use lemon water to gargle. Those with kidney stones should use a lot of lemons.

GINGER: Ginger has a warming effect and, stimulates circulation. If added in cooking or in making energy soup, it will counteract the "coldness" of some foods. In cooking, it is best used by midday. When used externally, it has the same warming effect. To use, grate a handful of ginger, wrap in cheese cloth, and boil in water for ten to fifteen minutes. Dip washing cloth in ginger water and apply on any area of the body that needs a little stimulation. For common colds and sniffles, apply to the chest. For weak kidneys, apply to the lower back. Even ringing in the ears can be relieved by applying a ginger compress to the kidney area for half an hour.

MOLASSES: It is the by-product of making white sugar. Sugar cane is actually a grass, nutritious if eaten whole. In the making of white sugar, all the nutritious parts, vitamins and minerals are concentrated in the molasses, including vanadium. Vanadium can help the breakdown of cholesterol. Those with high cholesterol can take one tablespoonful of molasses per day.

MISO: There are many varities of miso, made of soybeans, barley, buckwheat, or rice. It is rich in vitamin B12, one of the best sources for vegetarians. Miso also contains an enzyme that can help the body eliminate radioactive compounds. During the Second World War, when the atomic bomb was dropped on Hiroshima, the people at the Macrobiotic hosptial survived. The director told everyone to take miso straight, immediately after the bombing. The Catholic hospital next door had many casualties. In order to utilize the enzyme, add miso just before serving. It can replace salt or soy sauce for seasoning.

SEA VEGETABLES: Sea vegetables are good sources of minerals. Modern agricultural practices use chemical fertilizers; thus, the soil can easily be deficient in trace minerals. One can replenish these from the ocean. Lack of minerals can cause many illnesses.

KIDNEY-TONIC SOUP: Cook equal amounts of black beans, black dates, peanuts, wintermelon skin and molasses in water until soft. This is good for strengthening the kidneys. One can use this several times per week.

Houston, 1987

Chapter 16
The Use of Edible Weeds

A few years ago, I read a book written by an eighty year old doctor: "Nature's Healing Grasses." I became aquainted with medicinal uses of weeds, including dandelion, comfrey, nettle, seaweed and lambs quarter. Each of these weeds have their special use. Not only is their nutritional value high, but because of their deep roots they contain many minerals. Weeds also do not have pesticides. This doctor has sucessfully treated diabetes, arthritis, and cancer with weeds. The way these weeds were used in making green drink: blenderize all these kinds of greens in one cup of pineapple juice.

Besides the weeds mentioned above, purseland is often used. In Hunan, it is dried to treat diarrhea. Dried purseland can be used in cooking, and is quite flavorful. Dr. Ann Wigmore of Boston used fresh purseland to treat Bursitis. Purseland can be eaten fresh, cooked or dried.

Dandelion has very deep roots, and therefore contains rich sources of minerals, in particular calcium. One fourth-generation doctor of Chinese medicine uses dandelions to treat stomach cancer with good results. Both the leaves and roots can be used. The tender greens can be eaten in salad, and the roots boiled to make tea.

Aloe Vera does not belong in the category of backyard weeds but it was also originally a weed. It has many uses, from healing wounds, to burns, ulcers, constipation and diabetes. It facilitates the elimination of waste matter from the intestine. It can remove parasites if enough is taken. Those with poor digestion can take it in the morning, or before going to bed. It cleanses not only the intestinal tract but also the stomach, liver, kidney, spleen, and bladder. It helps in cases of menstration blockage.

Besides these common weeds, each region has its own special ones. In 1984 I returned to Taiwan for a visit. I had the fortune to visit the Hua-Liang sugar station and tasted a variety of weeds. Some were stir-fried, others marinated. There were at least four types. The memory of the fragrance still remains, even though I do not remember their names.

Weeds are cheap, delicious and nutritious, with fewer concerns about pesticides. Weeds should be identified and used.

Houston, 1987

Chapter 17
On the Treatment of
Some Chronic Diseases

DIABETES: This is a condition in which the pancreas is not secreting enough insulin, resulting in blood sugar being too high. If not taken care of properly, in later stages it will cause impaired eye-sight and wounds that will not heal. Diabetes usually begins with weakening of the digestive tract. To reverse the condition, start eating foods that are easily digested. All the foods introduced in the book belong to this category. Avoid greasy and refined products such as cakes and cookies. Eat more fresh fruits and vegetables, especially those containing high levels of potassium, thus stimulating the secretion of insulin.

HIGH BLOOD PRESSURE: The most common cause of high blood pressure is too much sodium in the diet. Eating potassium-rich vegetables and fruits will lower the blood pressure. Another cause is weakening of the kidneys or too much stress. Excess intake of protein and stress can cause high blood pressure.

GALLSTONE: Gallstones are usually caused by overeating, and too rich a diet, in particular fat, sugar and refined flour products. Those who do not like to drink water also have higher risks of getting gallstones. Medications for reducing blood pressure also increase the chances of getting gallstones. People over twenty usually have some stones. If the stones are small, people at most have only the symptom getting gas after a meal. Once one feels pain in the liver area, it is already quite serious. The method of removal is as follows: Drink four glasses of apple juice or eat four to five apples daily for five days. Eat normally. The apple juice or fruit softens the stones. On the sixth day, skip dinner. In the evening at six take one Tbsp. of Epsom salt in one glass of warm water. Repeat at eight. At ten in the evening, mix half a glass of olive oil and half a glass of lemon juice and drink. The stones come out in the stool on the seventh day. Look for them in the stool, green in color.

ALLERGIES: Allergies are caused by lack of B vitamins and minerals. The sources of B vitamins are yeast and sprouts. Minerals can be gotten from molasses, bran, whole grains and sea vegetables.

ARTHRITIS: This condition can be improved with mineral supplements. In the U.S. there are reports of improvement from arthritis by taking alfalfa tablets and barley green powder. Both of these foods are rich in minerals and trace minerals.

CANCER: There are articles focused entirely on the subject. In the natural treatment of cancer, enema plays an important role. It facilitates the elimination of toxic waste from the body. Coffee enema and wheatgrass implants are both good.

PIMPLES, SKIN RASHES: The skin is one of the paths for elimination. If the large intestine and the lungs are unable to completely eliminate wastes, then wastes can come through the skin. Usually individuals with strong metablism have the energy to eliminate through the skin. To soothe the skin, use fresh lemon juice or finely ground oatmeal paste. If the skin is itchy, the oatmeal paste is best. The diet should be light, free of oily and sugary food. One can also drink barley water. The British Royalties use this method to keep the skin smooth. Usually one year after the change of diet, some of the body waste will come out through the skin. This is normal.

FEVER AND HEADACHES: Most people will have fever or headaches from time to time. If this is caused by eating stale food or greasy food, take a coffee enema first. Then drink fresh lemon juice in warm water to speed the excretion of the poison.

DIARRHEA: Occassional diarrhea is caused by getting a cold, or eating bad food. Use a coffee enema first, and then eat thin oatmeal. If it is chronic, lasting one week or several months, the causes can be due to air pollution. According to Chinese medicine, large intestine and lungs are energetically connected. Avoid going out too much and drink plenty of rejuvelac to stimulate the elimination of poison. White fungus is also helpful to the lungs. Goldenseal root powder can be used for diarrhea caused by infection.

Chapter 18
Casual Conversation on Cancer Treatment

The word "cancer" usually elicits a strong emotional reaction, and is not a subject for casual conversation. So, why this choice of the title?

Firstly, worrying interferes with good health, especially those with sickness. "Casual conversation" encourages a lighter atmosphere.

Secondly, the treatments discussed are not conventional surgery, radiation and chemotherapy.

Thirdly, these treatments although effective, have not been tested in large scale clinical trials. They are merely experiential. Cancer is an illness that can be prevented and treated. If the medical community and the public had a correct understanding of the illness, then there would not be so much fear surrounding the disease, preventing also much unnecessary suffering and expense.

In both prevention and treatment of cancer, one must be aware of both the psychological and physical aspects, external and internal factors.

Let us start with prevention. The National Academy of Sciences recently published a report on cancer prevention. The conclusion is that aside from alcohol and smoking, food and cancer have the strongest link. For example, one study found that if smokers regularly eat carrots, the incidence of cancer is lower than for smokers who do not eat carrots. Carrots are rich in vitamin A, a cancer-inhibiting nutrient. Dark leafy greens are also protective against cancer. There are several recommendations for prevention of cancer: reduce oil, fat, salt and sugar consumption; increase consumption of fresh vegetables, fruits, and whole grains. These recommendations are based on numerous scientific studies. The details will not be given here.

Of course, environmental and physiological factors are important in the onset of cancer. However there are also psychological factors. This observation is at least 1000 years old. Chinese medicine has for thousands of years understood the relationship between emotions and diseases. To have little desire is a way to keep healthy. This includes moderation in food and simplicity of life style. In the Western medical tradition there is also literature on the relation between cancer and emotions. Dr. Galen wrote in 200 B.C. that women of melancholy disposition are more prone to breast cancer. This was based on his medical experience. There are a lot of modern day studies showing this. Long term depression combined with lack of a warm childhood can put one at high risk for cancer. Often one to two years before the onset of cancer, the patients have lost interest in living or hope for the future, or have experienced major stress and change in life. This can be loss of a spouse or other major changes. Unhappiness can impair many body functions, especially immune function. Because cancer can be caused by many factors, one should be aware of all these different factors in prevention.

The treatments discussed here are "folk" medicine. The main difference from hospital treatment is that the method is mild, with no side-effects. Those without sickness or with other chronic illnesses can all benefit. The result? There are many successful cases, and the news spreads by word of mouth. No treatment is going to be 100% successful, but at least it will improve the sick person's constitution. Each of the three treatments listed below have their strengths, and can be practiced together: food therapy; Chi Gong; and herbal medicine.

1. Food therapy:

In the discussion on cancer prevention, the importance of food was already mentioned. The most basic for those with cancer is that the food should at least be consistent with the principal of prevention: that is low fat, high fiber, ample fresh fruits and vegetables, and reduction of salt and sugar.

In recent years food therapy is becoming better known in the U.S.. The first involves the use of raw food: carrots, sprouts, cucumber, celery, spinach, parsley, etc. and seasonal fruits. Other recommended foods are nuts, sesame seeds, sunflower seeds and wheatsprouts. This school of thought is mainly from the Hippocrates Health Institute. It has been established for twenty years. Dr. Ann Wigmore, the founder and director has written many books on the subject. The most detailed is "Be Your Own Doctor." Her story is described in Chapter twelve "Let Your Body Be Your Own Doctor." Another book entitled, "How I Conquered Cancer Naturally," was written by Edie Mae, based on her experiences at H.H.I.. She had breast cancer, but controlled it entirely through a change of diet. This food therapy avoids meat, fish, sea food, white rice, white flour products, white sugar, and canned goods. Steamed and quickly stir-fried food can be used.

The second food therapy is called "Macrobiotics," introduced to the U.S. through Michio Kushi. This food therapy is based on Eastern tradition, with over twenty years of history in the U.S.. The diet emphasizes balance of yin and yang. Extreme yang food such as meat and extreme yin food such as sugar can easily throw the body out of balance. Sickness is the result of the body being out of balance. Grains are neutral, so are vegetables.

One can eat a lot without going out of balance. Macrobiotic ways of eating emphasize eating of seasonal food and food grown locally. People living in temperate zones should not eat food grown in the tropical zone, and in winter one should not eat summer food.

Macrobiotic food has benefited people with cancer. One music professor from the Midwest had a cancerous tumor of the pancreas the size of a fist. The tumor dissolved after adoption of the diet and did not recur in seven years. Later he died of hepatitis, and the doctor obtained proof that the cancer had disappeared. The cause of his death was related to the biopsy he first had.

Another book, based on the experience of Anthony J. Sattilaro, M.D., President of Methodist Hospital, entitled "Recalled by Life," was written with Tom Monte. The book is based on the author's being diagnosed as having cancer and by chance learning of food therapy, from May 1978 to the summer of 1981. Dr. Sattilaro was diagnosed as having prostate cancer in 1978. The X-rays showed that the cancer had spread to the bones in the head, shoulder, chest, and spine. He was forty-seven, at the peak of his career, and just promoted to be president of the Hospital. The illness changed everything. The survival rate for people getting this cancer before fifty is very low, the most optimistic prediction is that he would live three years, maybe not even eighteen months. Both surgery and hormone treatment did not halt the spread of cancer.

Just as he was preparing for his end, his father died of cancer. On the way back from the funeral, he was discouraged, to say the least. He picked up two hitch-hikers, a rather out of character gesture for him. In the car one fell asleep and the other talked about studying natural food therapy in Boston. When the young man found out Sattilaro had cancer, his said: "Cancer is not difficult to treat." To a doctor this is merely the enthusiastic ignorance of the youth. The young man continued sincerely that proper food can reverse cancer, and promised to send him some literature. A few weeks later he received a book documenting the reversal of cancer with diet: A Macrobiotic Approach to Cancer. From this beginning, with the attitude that nothing would be lost by trying, he overcame cancer completely in five years. For a doctor steeped in the Western medical training to accept the whole theory of yin-yang and disease is very difficult. Only his own personal experience convinced him.

The Macrobiotic diet is completely different from Dr. Sattilarao's former diet. He was a single medical doctor who ate three meals a day at restauarnts. He would have meat at every meal, and deserts at dinner, sometimes even a second helping. Although he had had stomach problem for over twenty years, he ignored them and took medications. According to the guidelines of the Macrobiotic diet, he was to avoid meat, fish, all animal products, oil, sugar, and flour products. His diet was 50% brown rice, 25-30% vegetables, 15% beans and sea vegetables, and some miso soup. Also he was not to overeat, and not to go to bed with a full stomach. Every mouthful had to be well chewed. After one month, his health started to improve. The back pain of over twenty years stopped. After fifteen months he went back for X-rays; all the cancerous growth had vanished. His digestive problems of over twenty years also vanished. He hoped others can benefit from his experience, and ordered the hospital to offer brown rice and vegetables. He also began a study to observe other cancer patients' response to the Macrobiotic diet. Additional note: vegetables can be steamed or boiled. Those without cancer can use a small amount of oil for stir-frying.

2. Chi Gong:

In the eyes of many Chinese, there is an aura of mystery surrounding Chi Gong. Some think of it in the same terms as

Kung Fu and aerobics. In fact, Chi Gong is an ancient Chinese medical art, mentioned in the classic on Chinese medicine "The Yellow Emperor's Text on Internal Medicine," and placed in the top place, above acupuncture and herbal medicine. Using Chi Gong to treat illnesses has many advantages, it is inexpensive, painless and beneficial regardless of whether there is illness. Chi Gong was still very popular in the Han dynasty. In the 1000 year old Han tomb discovered in Hunan, many medical texts were found. Among these were found extensive drawings on Chi Gong. Later in history, Chi Gong lost its place in medicine and became more associated with Kung Fu and Taoist practice.

In recent years, Chi Gong has been enjoying a revival of interest in China, mainly for medical purpose. This "new" Chi Gong is beneficial for all kinds of illnesses. The main one is a walking form. The mind is relaxed and made optimistic first. To help the mind become still, one can choose a theme to focus on, such as a nearby flower or tree. Whenever distracting thoughts come, return the thought to the theme. For most chronic illnesses, one hour a day is sufficient for improvement of health. Cancer patients need to practice four hours. The best environment for practice is morning in the forest, particularly a pine forest. The walking form is like that of a walk, with the heel touching the ground first and then the the whole foot. Both arms swing easily back and forth. For cancer patients, it is most important to breathe in lots of oxygen. The breath is two inhalations and one exhalation. One usually starts with the left foot. The whole body should be relaxed and "rounded." The eyes look straight ahead. Besides the walking form, there is preparation, and closing. In accordance to one's physical condition, there are over twenty different types of Chi Gong. There are now over 7000 cases of cancer patients recovering from their illnesses. These include lung cancer patients and those with advanced stages of cancer. I met two lung cancer patients who recovered through Chi Gong.

The basis for Chi Gong's therapeutic benefit is related to the fact that Chi Gong stimulates the blood and Chi circulation. This comes through relaxation of the body and mind and physical movement combined with breathing. Making sound is another aspect of Chi Gong. Depending on the physical condition, one can make different sounds. At the minimum, Chi Gong can improve one's emotional state, sleep and digestion. If cancer patients are taking chemotherapy or radiation, then Chi Gong can reduce the effects from these treatments.

One needs a good teacher to learn Chi Gong. However there is a simple exercise, a kind of Chi Gong. It is called the hand swing exercise. According to legend, this came from Bodhidharma, the first Zen patriarch. Stand with both feet parallel to the shoulder. Tighten the lower body, with the toes gripping the floor. Tighten also the rectal muscles. Relax the upper body, with the tongue touching the upper palate. Allow the arms to relax and push backwards, about thirty degree, then let go. Count each push as one. Beginners can do 100 to 200 times, increasing to 1000 times. In Taiwan there are also cases of cancer patients recovering from this exercise. My aunt is one of them.

3. Herbal Medicine

The use of herbs in medicine has thousands of years of history in China. The legendary first doctor in Chinese history, Shen-Nung tasted 100 different plants to identify different herbal medicines. That herbs are effective in cancer is not a new discovery. Chinese doctors find the appropriate medicine for each person. The general approach is to strengthen the body and expel the wastes. For example, although there is one disease called cancer, the causes can be many; therefore the herbal medicines are many too. Some are particularly beneficial: there are scientific studies which show that white fungus, Angelic root, and Neu tsen tse increase the immune function. It is best to consult an experienced Chinese medical doctor for the specific uses of these herbs.

The use of herbs in other countries has also enjoyed a long history. The better known ones for treating cancer are: Chaparral among American Indians, and Red Clover Blossom among Gypsies. The use of these herbs by themselves is sometimes enough. One 86 year old man in Utah had a cancerous growth on his face. He refused surgery. After drinking Chaparral tea for eight months, he recovered. His doctor tried it on himself with good results and also used it on other patients with good result. Jethro Kloss in "Back to Eden" talks about the use of Red Clover Blossom in the treatment of cancer. One can simmer it for 15 minutes. Mr. Kloss, in the chapter on cancer treatment, mentioned, besides herbal medicine, the need for simple natural food, fresh air, sunshine, water and skin massages.

The above mentioned herbs although beneficial when used alone, sometimes produce amazing results when used together. Jason Winters wrote of his battle with cancer in the book "Killing Cancer." He discovered by chance the combination of three herbs (two of which are Chaparral and Red Clover Blossom; the third is unidentified) which cured him of throat cancer. The story is as follows: four years ago Mr. Winters discovered that he had cancer of the throat. Just the initial biopsy took six hours on the operating table. The doctor told him he had three months to live. He accepted radiation but refused surgery. The doctors were going to remove his tongue and throat muscles but did not guarantee extending his life. In order to find an ancient Oriental herb, he went to Singapore. From an old lady in a village he found the Asian herb. He took it everyday. Although the growth stopped, it did not regress. Next he went to England and learned of Red Clover Blossom. He added that to this daily drink. But his body continiued to weaken everyday. After he used up his savings he went home and kept up with the daily intake of Asian and European herb and added Chaparral. He boiled them separately but did not improve much. One day when he was at the lowest point, he mixed all three and drank them together. A miracle happened. He could feel that this was exactly what he needed. He drank 16 cups. After that his health started to improve. Within three weeks, the cancer had completely disappeared. He returned to work after nine weeks. When the news got out, hundreds of people would line up to seek out the herbs. One minister drank it with good result, curing himself of hemorrhoids of twenty years duration. There are over 30,000 people who have tried the herbal mixture. In the world there are over one million that have tried. Thousands of letters testify to the benefit.

CONCLUSION:

Cancer is caused by many factors. In the treatment one should also approach it from different angles. The most important is to help the person regain the body's defense system. The methods mentioned here are all gentle without side effects.

"Sickness comes through the mouth" is particularly appropriate in the case of cancer. The prevention and treatment of cancer should begin with food. Food can improve the body, while herbs and Chi Gong can further strengthen the recovery. If the three can be combined, the result is best.

To overcome cancer, the patient must make the determination to fight the illness. If one is unsure and half-hearted, one will not achieve the desired result. One's lifestyle should be changed, too. Smokers should quit and take time to exercise. "Arm swinging" or Tai Chi Chuan are suited for those who have a weak constitution. The last point is to have a positive outlook on life.

Appendix:

I became interested in cancer while a student in college. I collected information on the disease. Later, when I went to M.I.T. for doctoral study of chemistry, I had the opportunity to visit the Hippocrates Health Institute of Boston. During those four years I learned much about living food. After receiving my doctorate degree, I decided to enter cancer research at the University of Texas Cancer Center. My initial studies found that wheatgrass is capable of inhibiting the activation of carcinogens. Later chlorophyll was identified to be the active factor. All chlorophyll containing vegetables have inhibiting activity against carcinogens. Later my research focused on biophysics, discovering the electropotential of rat liver tumors to be lower than that of normal liver. This was related to the low content of oxygen in cancerous tissue.

Between September and December of 1981, under the auspices of the U.S. National Academy of Sciences, I went to Beijing to study the relation between diet and esophagus cancer in Henan, Linxian. This experience further convinced me of the importance of diet in the prevention of cancer. During three months in Beijing, I met Madame Guo Ling, the famous Chi Gong master. I realized cancer is indeed curable, but one must address both the physical and emotional levels. In 1982 after leaving China, I went to Holland for six months to continue my research. I learned about food therapy promoted there by Dr. Moerman, using an approach similar to the raw food therapy described earlier. Unfortunately this old doctor did not speak English and I did not speak Dutch, so we could not communicate.

Since going into cancer research, I have often received letters from people suffering from cancer. They know that my approach is different than the conventional approach. When they have exhausted all options, they write to me. I had an aunt who used to live in Taipei. In 1975 she got cancer, and it had spread to three places. Her depression is understandable. I told her about the raw food therapy. In a short time her appetite and digestion improved, and the tumors began to decrease in size. After eight months, she started "Arm swing" exercise and within one month there was no more sign of cancer. Seven years later she moved to the U.S. to be with her daughters. She is healthy at the time of this writing.

Cancer is curable. I wish the news to be known to more people. This is the motivation for writing this article.

Houston, 1984

Chapter 19
Further Conversation on Cancer Treatment in the Nineties

Five years after writing "Casual Conversation on Cancer Therapy," my basic approach to cancer remains unchanged. The only difference is more experience and additional information, particularly in relation to the emotional and spiritual factors in the development of sickness.

In November of 1989, I visited Grenoble, France and learned about a cancer treatment center focused on the psychological aspects of cancer. The center utilizes the approach discovered by Dr. R.G. Hamer, a German doctor based in Cologne. Patients are helped through talking, and resolving inner conflicts and shocks. Dr. Hamer has found that inner conflicts and shocks are the main trigger that sets off cancer. In 1979 after his son was murdered, both he and his wife came down with cancer. He was a specialist in cancer; the experience taught him that cancer can be triggered through the mind, and the development stage can be very short. He reversed his own cancer after resolving his inner conflicts. He discovered that his patients also experienced some form of shock or inner conflict combined with inability to talk about it (or had no one who would listen) before the onset of cancer. The patients were helped through talking it out and through finding specific solutions to the problem. Depending on the nature of the shock or conflict, lesions in the brain would appear, followed by the detection cancer in the corresponding organs. For example, cancer of the left breast is related to conflict between mother and child. The right side is related to conflict with others. Cancer of the colon is related more to "territorial" conflict at work, such as areas of responsibility and control. Cancer of the lung is more related to fear of death; liver with anger, bitterness and resentment. Over all he collected 10,000 cases.

In the treatment of cancer, Dr. Hamer uses the approaches of talking, letting the patient talk it out, and of resolving conflicts. I met a woman in France with cancer of both breasts which had metastasized throughout the body. Before the onset of disease, one of her sons has tried to commit suicide, one had had an explosion at home, and the third son had also had problems. Then she had a fight with her husband. Soon afterwards she developed cancers in both breasts that spread throughout the body.

As the saying goes: "In life, eight or nine times out ten things do not go as we wish." When conflicts or problems arise, it is important not to repress. Whenever possible, talk it out among friends and family. If it is a situation or problem without a ready-made solution, one can use the method of thought transformation to face it. Some of the folk sayings of China are really the wisdom of thousands of years: "lose money, reduce trouble," "life and death have their own courses, riches and positions are up to heaven." If one understands karma, one would realize: "You harvest squash if you planted seeds of squash, and harvest beans after planting beans." To have all go well, one must "refrain from all evil, do all that is good." At the same time one should repent past wrong doings. Further, life is like a dream; everything is changing all the time. What is the use of getting stuck on the sharp end of the horns of the bull? What is the use of getting overwhelmed with anger? Think, where are the heros of the bygone days? One will calm down after thinking things through. At the same time, one should accumulate as much positive energy as possible, helping others in whatever way one can. To extend one's life, it is important to not kill, and to save as many lives as possible. The number saved should be at the least same as one's age; the more the better.

A Canadian woman more than five years ago had advanced melanoma, which spread to the lungs. The doctors told her she had three months to live, without any hope. Under such circumstances, she decided to die in a beautiful place, such as Nepal. There she met a high Lama in the Himalayas through a friend. The Lama was Zopa Rinpoche, who told her to save as many lives as possible. After her return to Vancouver, she went to the dock everyday and bought live fish and shrimp and put them back in the ocean. She also saved dogs and cats that were going to be killed. After four months, her cancer disappeared completely. Last year when I talked to her over the phone, she told me three month ago her cancer returned to her left breast. She repeated the same, becoming a strict vegetarian and saving lives. Again the cancer disappeared. I asked her how many lives she saved everyday. She replied: "One hundred on the average." Besides liberating animals, she also took time to walk, reflecting on the purpose of her life. After the sickness, she changed profession from fashion design consulting to environmental protection and ethics and compassion in business.

Florida, 1990

Chapter 20
The Application of Chinese Traditional Medicine

I have received in total, six years of Chinese education in Taiwan, four years in grade school and two years in middle school. Perhaps that is why I have a fascination for traditional Chinese heritage, in particular Chinese traditional medicine. Living in the U.S. provided very little opportunity to study. In the fall of 1981, under the auspices of U.S. China scholarly exchange program, I went to Beijing, China to study the relation between esophagus cancer and diet. I lived in China for three months. During this period, not only my Chinese became more fluent, but also I encountered Chi Gong, Chinese medicine, and acupressure with mung beans. My first teacher in Chinese medicine was Doctor Yao, a fourth generation Chinese medical doctor. His grandfather used to treat the Empress Dowager. He was living in seclusion, not meeting visitors. Through a friend's introduction, he accepted my request to study Chinese medicine. From then on every Friday afternoon I went to his home to receive teaching on basic theory in Chinese medicine, and then stayed for dinner. After two or three months I had a basic understanding of Chinese medicine. Dr. Yao put the emphasis on history of Chinese medicine and major medical writings. The rest he felt I could later look up and read in the texts on my own. He especially had a lot of experience treating cancer. He had written down generations of experience on cancer treatment in a book. Unfortunately during the cultural revolution, the manuscript was taken from him and has never been found again. Also during the cultural revoultion, ten roomsful of medical texts, kept in the family for generations were burned. He was heart broken, and this is one of the main reasons why he is living as a recluse. From Dr. Yao, I understood why Chinese medicine cannot be tested in Western clinical trials. The basis of Chinese medicine is treating the person, and not the symptom. Two people with the same disease may require different medicine because of different causes and conditions. One medicine may cure one person, but may not be suited for someone else with the same disease. To investigate Chinese medicine, one cannot transplant the western medical approach to studying it.

Moved by curiosity, I also took up the study of Chi Gong and acupressure with mung beans. Through these I learned of the depth and preciousness of Chinese traditional medicine. Chi Gong taught me the existence of Chi and meridians. Acupressure with mung beans also showed me the miraculous healing power of traditional medicine.

Acupressure with mung beans comes from ear acupuncture. At that time, every Sunday in Ditan Park, two or three hundred people would line up to have their ears "beaned" by Mr. Wang and his assistants. Mr. Wang's grandfather is a Chinese medical doctor. His official work is connected with the military. Treating people with mung beans is an interest and labor of love. He has an amazing ability to diagnose, by merely looking at a person's ears, a person's entire medical history. He is usually right on target.

The beans are first split in half, the flat side taped to a small square of surgical tape, and the round side pressed against the surface of the ear. It was amusing to see the individuals walking out of the park with white tapes all over their ears. It was a unique phenomenon of Ditan Park. The Chinese still prefer Chinese traditional medicine. But a shortage of Chinese doctors accounts for the large number of people coming to the park for medical treatment.

Mr. Wang gave many evening lectures on the theory of ear acupressure. Anyone was welcome. There were usually thirty people squeezed in a small room and sitting on benches. The electricity in the area was quite unpredictable. I always carried my flashlight to shine on the black board whenever the lights went out. Because the method of ear acupressure with mung beans is simple and without side effects, many beginners after one month were having success treating people. The students progressed very fast with the combination of learning theory in the classroom and hands-on experience in the park. I spent many Sundays observing. One elderly lady came with a stiff arm. After having a few beans in her ears, she could lift up her arm. In addition to treating the specific points, one always put beans in the areas corresponding to liver, spleen, kidneys. For all those with chronic diseases, these organs are weak. After the beans are pressed in place, one puts pressure on them several times a day, and keeps them in place for six days. This is one treatment phase. Depending on the condition, one can remove them at the end of six days or start the second round of six days after a few days of break.

The ears are connected to the whole body through the nervous system and through the Chi pathways or meridans (see graph 1). From the ears that one can see the condition of the entire body, and can affect the whole body. Old sickness shows up as scars or white spots. New diseases show up as red spots, purplish or excess blood vessels. Any unusual markings or scalings indicate problems in the corresponding area. In the beginning, one may not be able to tell. But experience is the best teacher. Look into the ears of friends and family members, especially those with a diagnosis of their physical condition. Learn what condition produces what symptoms in the ears.

The basics of Chinese medicine will be introduced below to facilitate the ear diagnosis. An ear chart and the corresponding areas are shown. The sensitive points in the ears can be detected with a pinhead touching the skin. If one gets a feeling of electricity or heat, then one can put beans on that point. One can also use a hair pin or yarn needle to find sensitive points.

The major difference between Chinese culture and Western culture is that the former is more right-brain oriented. The right brain is characterized by intuition, wholistic, inspirational and artistic qualities, while the left brain is characterized by logical and partial processes. Many of the world problems we face are the result of logical and partial approaches to solving problems, neglecting the whole. The traditional Chinese medical system is the product of right brain; therefore it has its special contribution to modern medicine.

To study Chinese medicine, one first needs to understand meridians. Meridians are energetic pathways for the flow of Chi, distributed throughout the body. There are twelve main pathways, and two master ones named Governor and Conception, which control the entire 12 Yang and Yin meridians. There are eight extra meridians outside of these. In Chi Gong practices, the focus is often on balancing the Chi in the eight extra meridians. The key role they play is in communications between other main meridians. Often physical problems are the result of communication; one part is lacking while the other has excess energy. Of the 12 meridians, those distributed in the front are Yin meridians, and those in the back are Yang meridians. Six meridians terminate in the fingers, and six in the toes. They are symmetrically on the right and left side and equal in Yang and Yin meridians. Please see graph 2 for more details.

LUNG meridian (yin) terminates in the thumb. Besides the lungs, the attribute under its influence is skin. Grief and sadness will affect the lung meridian. LARGE INTESTINE (yang) meridian begins at the index finger, and forms a pair with the lung meridian. Problems in the large intestine will indirectly affect the lungs. The reverse is also true. For example, for a period of one month Houston had severe air pollution. Many people had diarrhea problems. Without the understanding of Chi and meridians, it would be difficult to explain. The pollution directly affected the lungs, but indirectly the large intestine.

CIRCULATION meridian (yin) terminates at the middle finger and controls blood pressure and circulation. TRIPLE HEATER (yang) begins at ring finger and controls hormonal system and energy level. Those who are tired all the time usually have imbalance in the triple heater meridian.

HEART meridian (yin) terminates on the inside of the little finger. Overexcitment and inability to express joy all have a negative effect on the heart meridian. SMALL INTESTINE meridian (yang) begins at the outside of the small finger, and forms a pair with the heart meridian. The ability of the small intestine to absorb nutrients affects blood formation, indirectly affecting the health of the heart.

We will continue by discussing the meridians that terminate at the toes: SPLEEN meridian (yin) begins at the outside of the big toe. It includes the pancreas function. Besides blood sugar level, the flesh (loss or gain) are influenced by the spleen meridian. One of the first symptoms of sickness is the loss of flesh; this is related to the functioning of the spleen. Obsessive thinking and worrying weaken the spleen.

LIVER meridian (yin) begins at the inner part of the big toe, in control of tendons, nails and eyes. Pain in the tendons is often due to liver problems. One of the early signs of cancer is tendon and muscle pains. The liver is an important organ for elimination of waste from the body. Those with chronic illnesses will have a weak liver. The condition of the nails, especially the big toe nails is indicative of the liver condition. If the nail bulges out, is broken, or the color darkens, that indicates some problem with the liver. Usually when the nail bulges out or is ingrown, it is due to eating too much concentrated protein. Meat and eggs all belong to this category. If the diet is changed to vegetables and grains, the problem with the nails will improve. Some cancer patients undergoing chemotherapy will find the toe nails to be in a bad state. It is because of the damage of drugs on the liver. The liver is closely connected with anger. When the "liver fire" is high (a Chinese expression for volatile temperament), it is due to imbalance in the liver meridian; therefore one is easily provoked. The breasts are also connected with the liver meridian. Some recent medical studies have found that women who develop breast cancer tend to repress their anger. Repressed anger harms the liver and the breasts. Appropriate expression of anger and emotions is important to health.

STOMACH meridian (yang) ends on the second and third toes. It is a pair with the spleen meridian. The stomach meridian controls digestion and energy or aliveness. Poor digestion can indirectly affect the spleen meridian, causing diabetes.

GALL BLADDER meridian (yang) ends on the fourth toe, and is a pair with the liver meridian. Imbalance in the gall bladder can bring about frequent headaches. Gallstones are another symptom; one can consult chapter 23 of this book about using apple juice to flush out gallstones.

KIDNEY meridian (yin) begins at the inside of the little toe, forming a pair with the bladder meridian. In Chinese medicine, the kidney meridian plays an important role in the body. The meridian system includes adrenal glands, bones, teeth, ears, hearing, and hair on the head. It also affects the quality of our sleep. When the kidney meridian is not in balance, one can have ringing in the ears, loss of hair, no energy, nightmares, and restless sleep. The kidneys are vulnerable to cold. The habit of taking a cold drink is very bad for the kidneys. When the icy liquid enters the stomach, it cools the stomach and then the kidneys, just behind the stomach. Those suffering from ringing in the ears can apply a hot ginger compress to the back for 30 minutes. Often once is enough to stop the ringing. There are many ways to strengthen the kidneys; the most important is to avoid salt and animal protein. Black colored foods such as black beans, black dates, and sea weeds are all beneficial to the kidneys. The emotion of fear weakens the kidneys. Conversely when the kidneys are weak, one will be more fearful.

Lastly, we will discuss the BLADDER meridian (yang) which ends on the outside of the little toe. Its function is to regulate water. If out of balance, one will have difficulty urinating or will experience loss of control. Because it is a pair with the kidney meridian, if the kidney meridians are weak, the bladder may also be out of balance.

Chinese medicine has thousands of years of history. Even one lifetime is not enough to master it all. Only the very basic concepts are introduced here for the purpose of gaining understanding in the treatment of disease and improvement of health.

Houston, 1987

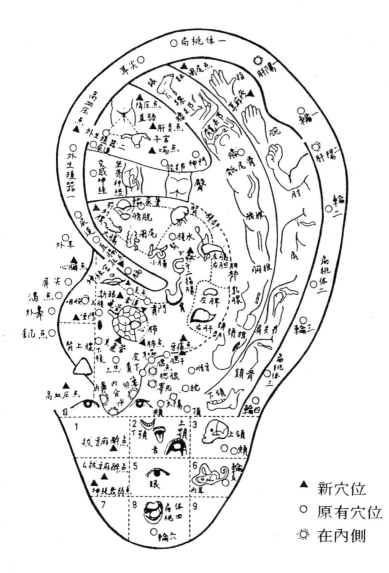

▲ 新穴位
○ 原有穴位
☼ 在內側

Graph One
Ear Acupressure Chart

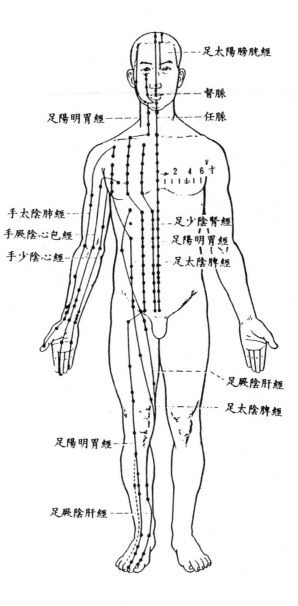

Graph 2-1
Fourteen Meridians (Front)

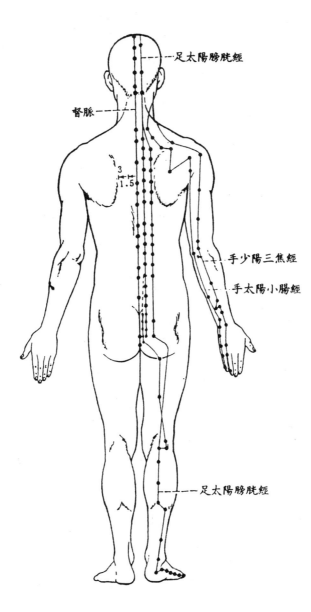

足太陽膀胱經

督脈

3
1.5

手少陽三焦經

手太陽小腸經

足太陽膀胱經

Graph 2-2
Fourteen Meridians (Back)

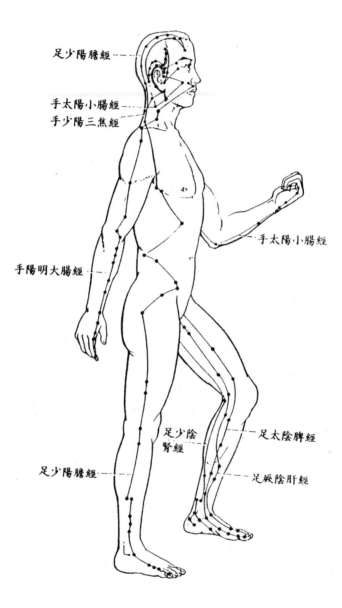

足少陽膽經

手太陽小腸經
手少陽三焦經

手太陽小腸經

手陽明大腸經

足少陰
腎經

足太陰脾經

足少陽膽經

足厥陰肝經

Graph 2-3
Fourteen Meridians (Side)

Chapter 21
Instinctual Nutrition - How to Choose What The Body Needs

In a suburb of Paris is a health center geared to teaching people to use their sense of smell to choose what their body needs. The founder, Guy Claude-Burger, is a physicist and a cellist. He has even performed in symphonies. Unfortunately at the age of 26 he developed cancer of the throat. He went to live in the forest to find a way to regain his health. This change of life helped him recover. Also he rediscovered our survival instinct, our sense of smell.

Actually, our earliest nutritionist was our nose and tongue. When we smelled foods that were needed, we would salivate. We would also find the food to be delicious. After we had had enough, the taste of the food would change. Sometimes the difference is in one bite. However, later with the introduction of food processing, heating and seasoning, our basic sense of smell and taste became very confused. We lost the ability to determine what our bodies needed. Even though we eat a lot, it is not necessarily what our body needs. It is no surprise that sickness follows.

In this health center near Paris, we are taught to relearn this instinct. All the foods provided are natural, and only those available on earth 10,000 years ago. They come from around the world, without heating and processing. At meal time, the foods are placed on several tables. The guests line up and smell each food item, sometimes using a small knife to break the skin to enhance the aroma. One first chooses the item that makes one's mouth water the most. Once the taste of that item loses its appeal, one then proceeds to the next food item that makes one's mouth water. This method of choosing and eating food, guided by one's sense of smell and taste, has helped some seriously ill people get well. If no food makes one's mouth water, it is possible the food one needs is not among the foods considered. Do not neglect unusual food. If one still does not find any food that makes one's mouth water, consider fasting for one meal. If it is so for several days, it indicates the digestive system needs resting; do not force feed.

For most people, the instinct for choosing food does not return immediately; continuing practice will help one improve. Due to the difference in body constitution, different people will require different food. Those born in the winter time have a more yin or "cold" constitution. They prefer cold food, salt, eggs, sugar, processed foods, soft and liquid foods. The recommendation for winter people is: eat less salt, avoid fasting, eat less of cold and raw food. Eat more root vegetables, naturally sweet vegetables, such as carrots, squash, sea vegetables, rice, millet and buckwheat, and hot soup with ginger. Those born in the spring likes sweets, milk products, fruits, salad, cakes and liquid. They should eat more of dried foods, dark green vegetables, less liquid, warm foods, quick stir-fried vegetables such as squash, brown rice, millet and buckwheat. Summer-born people like meat, sugar, alcohol, fruits, fried foods, salt and spices and tend to overeat. These people should eat more of the fresh raw vegetables, sour fruits, corn, barley, sea vegetables, white vegetables, less oil, and less food. Those born in the fall like simple food, salty taste, animal protein, coffee, bread and dry roasted food. These people should eat more variety, moist food, soup, sweet vegetables, and hot food. They should avoid cold drinks and cold food. Another important point is to take time to eat, chewing carefully. The above are recommendation from an expert in Chinese food therapy in the U.S..

It is emphasized again that because of an individual's living environment, and season of birth, one has different needs. To force the whole family to eat the same food is not advisable, especially with children. Children are best left to choose their own foods, excluding processed foods and "junk" foods.

Houston, 1987

Chapter 22
Food, Emotions and Personality

Most people are aware of the relationship between food and health. Less information is available on the impact of food on psychology. Actually this concept was known in ancient times. Mensius had said: "Meat-eaters are coarse," pointing out the effect of meat on spirituality. The tradition of Yoga from India has much to teach about the relation between food and mind. In Yoga the highest state in which to be is the state of stillness. To facilitate the achievement of that state, foods are recommdended that will help the mind to be clear and sharp. In this category are vegetables, legumes, grains, etc. Meat is not recommended because it tends to make the mind coarse, and not calm. Two psychologists (Drs. Saul and Jo Ann Miller) wrote a book in 1979 entitled: "Food for Thought, A New Look at Food and Behavior." The following are the essentials of the book.

The two authors have lived and worked on the North American Continent, Europe, and Asia, observing the relationship between food and behavior. They classified food as "expansive," "neutral," and "contractive." At the extreme end of expansive foods are drugs, alcohol, and sugar. At the extreme end of contractive foods are meats, fish, eggs, and cheese. Plant foods such as grains, seeds, vegetables and fruits are neutral, with the grains right at the center. Fruits are slightly on the side of expansive and seeds slightly on the side of contractive. How does this affect behavior? Fruits and vegetables make a person more expressive, open and interested in spiritual matters. One is more extroverted and optimistic. On the other hand, meat and fish make one more conservative, rigid, controlling, possessive, introverted and heavy. The neutral foods are helpful for one to be balanced in emotion and posture. The following are nine points in regard to food and behavior: 1. Expansive foods - open behavior. 2. Contractive food - conservative behavior. 3. Extreme diet - extreme behavior. 4. Neutral diet - balanced behavior. 5. Natural food - natural behavior. 6. Disintegrating food - disintegrating behavior. 7. Queer food - queer behavior. 8. High fat diet - reduced flow of energy, reduced energy and sensitivity. 9. Excess food - reduce sensitivity, energy and attractiveness.

The traditional foods of the East and West have always been based on grain. Modern American food is based predominantly on meat, egg, fruits, and vegetables. Sociologists in the fifties noted a general change in American personalities, from inwardly directed to outwardly directed. One lost the sense of self, being directed by outside opinions. The choice of food also became unbalanced. There is a four-fold increase in the use of processed food from 1910 to 1970. The increased use of processed food is the main cause of the change in psyche and body. On the average Americans consume 240 lbs of meat, 120 lbs of sugar, and 10 lbs of grains annually.

Extreme diet will bring about extreme behavior, extreme desire and thinking. Extreme diet will cause one to lose self-control; this is especially true of meat which stimulates sexual desires, but reduces sensitivity. Sugar makes one unrealistic, while reducing energy, making for strong sex drive but strange imagination. An unbalanced diet indirectly contributes to the spread of pornpographic literature and movies, and dissatisfaction in the relations between men and women.

The imbalance in diet not only brings about the extreme behavior mentioned above, but also increase criminal behavior. Although research in this area is limited, yet one can see the direct relation between the unbalanced diet and increase in crime in the U.S. and Europe. Low blood sugar has been linked with various criminal activities. A study in Argentina found among 129 criminals, only 13 had normal blood sugar level. In the Ohio report, among the 102 of those on probation, 82 had over 15 symptoms of low blood sugar. One even had over 50 symptoms. Once the diet is changed, cutting out sugar and refined starches, the behavior and attitude changes for the better. The best foods served in the jail are whole grains, fresh vegetables and fruits. This type of eating is best for helping criminals stay out of trouble.

We are originally in harmony with nature. Our "modern" life style can cause us to be separated from nature. One of the causes is eating in disconnection from nature. Traditional cultures have advised the use of seasonal food grown locally. With the advance of technology, those living in cold climates use heating systems, wear summer clothes indoors, and eat tropical foods such as oranges, bananas, sugar cane, and coffee. This causes us to be unprepared for living in the cold climate, forcing us to rely on heating, becoming like greenhouse plants, without resistance. On the other hand, those northerners who move to the south, still maintain the habits of the north, eating lots of meat. As a result they are unable to endure the heat of summer, requiring air conditioning and ice cold drinks. If one is aware of the environment in which one lives, one eats contractive food in the winter, such as grains, legumes, some animal products, and less fruits. Then one would not be bothered by the cold. In the summer if one eats fruits, salads and plant based protein, then one will not need air conditioning.

Lastly the emotional state of the cook can affect the food. Many cultures advise against eating food cooked by angry, sick or fearful persons. Eating food cooked by a loving person is very beneficial. Those who frequent restaurants are at the mercy of the chef's emotional state.

The above is a brief summary of the message in "Food for Thought," on the relation between diet and emotion.

Houston, 1987

Chapter 23
Case Studies

ULCER: A woman in Hawaii suffered from a stomach ulcer. X-rays showed the ulcerated area to be swollen. She could not eat fruits such as oranges. Following the suggestion of my mother, she started eating natural foods, and taking fresh comfrey leaf (taken on an empty stomach first thing in the morning). Within a few weeks, her condition improved. X-rays no longer showed inflammation and eating fruits did not bring pain.

ALLERGIES: An overseas Chinese in Australia suffered from hay fever for over ten years. Every pollen season she would suffer from difficulty of breathing. Taking Western medication made the condition worse. After taking one leaf of fresh comfrey everyday for one month, her allergy significantly improved. With greater confidence in the healing power of nature, she further changed her diet, increasing fruits and vegetables and decreasing meat. In the last ten years since the change in diet, her hay fever has not recurred and she is enjoying good health at the age of seventy. She even looks younger than before.

GALLSTONES: The cases of people removing gallstones with apple juice, epsom salt and olive oil are numerous. I know of seven cases, including myself. The following are a few examples:

Among my co-worker is a fifty year old tissue culturist named Jim. One day he complained of pain in the abdomen. Doctors suspected parasites. Despite taking medication for worms, he still suffered from pain, coupled with dizziness. I suggested it may be gallstones, and not parasites. Jim has been taking anti-cholesterolemic medication for several years. We checked and found one of the side effect of the medication is calcification of the bile duct. He followed the procedure for removing gallstones and passed many stones. His pain also went away.

Another case involves a secretary who suffered from gallstones. Doctors had recommended surgery, but she refused. She could not eat any greasy foods. She followed the instruction for removal of gallstones: four glasses of apple juice per day for five days. On the sixth day she took no dinner and took one Tbsp. of epsom salt at 6 p.m. and another at 8 p.m.. At 10 p.m. drank half a cup of olive oil mixed with half a cup of fresh lemon juice. Next morning around 7:30 a.m. she called with great excitement. She passed 14 stones, some as big as a thumb and others as fine as sand. From then on she could eat whatever she liked without effects.

A final case is a Chinese lady in her thirties living in Houston. Because of gallstones, she sometimes would be in pain four hours at a time. The doctor also urged surgery. She asked me for advice and I gave her the same remedy. She passed 20 to 30 stones the size of peas. My guess is that everyone has stones; the only difference is in the size and number.

LUNG CANCER: Lung cancer is very difficult to cure in the Western medical tradition. According to the U.S. National Cancer Institute, the five year survival rate is 10%. There is no difference in survival rate between those receiving treatment and no treatment. In May of this year a Chinese lung cancer patient came with his family to my office. He wanted to learn Chi Gong. In March he had been diagnosized with lung cancer. The doctors were going to operate immediately, but because he also had cancer of the large intestine, they removed that first. It was confirmed to be malignant. The lung surgery was postponed to

June. I suggested that he change his diet, and practice Waidan-gong. I gave him a copy of my article "Casual Conversation on Cancer Treatment." I also recommended taking Barley Green, and supplementing mineral intake with Goldstake. He started to practice Waidangong in early June, taking lesson from a graduate of the Taiwan International Instructors' training course. The day before his scheduled surgery in late June he went to M.D. Anderson for a checkup. They found that the tumor, originally measuring 1.5 cm, was almost gone. Surgery was cancelled. Since the doctors could not explain the reversal, they thought maybe it was a misdiagnosis for inflammation. The patient also did not tell the doctors of his other practices. Re-checking of his medical records showed that all X-rays and blood tests since March had indicated cancer. The only unknown was whether it was original or metastasized cancer. Only the test in June showed changes. I asked him and his family what he did during this period. They said he tried everything, so it is not clear which worked. To shrink lung cancer in less than two months is very remarkable. The integrated approach is most likely the reason for his quick recovery. Here is what he did: he consulted a Chinese doctor and took Chinese herbal medicine, ate a strict vegetarian diet, took barley green and mineral sup-plements, and practiced Waidangong.

Houston, 1987

Chapter 24
To Catch The "Spirit"
of "Flavor"

Translation note: The Chinese word for M.S.G., a flavor enhancer, is "Spirit of Flavor." This is a play on the word "spirit" which could mean essence or spirit as in "goblin" with an additional character added.

I left Taiwan to come to the U.S. at a young age. There was a period of twelve years during which I did not return to Taiwan. In 1984 I returned to Taiwan for a vacation. Unexpectedly, friends arranged for me to give public talks on the subject of cancer prevention. As part of the home-coming, there were also many invitations from friends to eat at vegetarian restaurants. After only a few days in Taiwan, I noticed tiredness and fogginess of the mind. This was rather unusual for me. I suspected it was due to the M.S.G. used in the restaurants. In order to fullfill all the speaking obligations, from then on I requested my hosts ahead of time: "Please, do not use M.S.G. in the food."

That visit to Taiwan allowed me to experience the effects of M.S.G.. I also heard many "theories" about M.S.G.. Some claimed it to be a "brain food." In order to gather the facts on M.S.G., I went to the library as soon as I returned to the U.S.. I searched through the literature about M.S.G., including its discovery, production and physiological effects in animal studies. I wrote an article on my findings and sent it to Taiwan. It never got published. Even the manuscript was lost. In 1992, I again visited Taiwan. M.S.G. was still widely used, especially in restaurants. Many people suffer from the side effects of M.S.G., but find it unavoidable when eating out. I thought to clarify the issue in regards to M.S.G. at the time of publication of my book.

The full name of M.S.G. is monosodium glutamate, formed by sodium and an amino acid, glutamine. The flavor comes from the amino acid. Glutamate is found in natural foods. We have it in our body, especially in our brain. It was discovered by a Japanese scientist who extracted it from a very flavorful seaweed. In the past, M.S.G. was a luxury item, few could afford it. Only in the last 20 or 30 years, as a result of inexpensive processes of production, M.S.G. is consumed in large quantities, especially in China and Southeast Asia. In the West, only some processed foods contain M.S.G.. Most people do not use it on a regular basis. It is not allowed in baby foods due to scientific studies showing that M.S.G. causes damage to the brain and visual nervous system of young animals such as chicks and mice.

Just how does M.S.G. affect us? It contains sodium and glutamate, therefore there are two effects. One is connected with the side effects of eating too much sodium: thirst, high blood pressure, and other problems associated with excessive sodium. Because M.S.G. is not salty, one can unknowningly consume too much sodium. Secondly glutamate functions as a neurotransmitter in the body. If one consumes it in concentrated form, it will interfere with the natural processes. Some individuals experience muscle paralysis, headaches, and even coma. Westerners normally do not use M.S.G.. The response from M.S.G. usually happens after eating at a Chinese restaruant. The medical name used for side effects from M.S.G. is "Chinese

restaurant syndrome." One out of four people is sensitive to
M.S.G.; women are more sensitive than men. Even one bowl of
wonton soup can bring on the symptoms, ranging from dizziness, headache, paralysis of facial muscle, tiredness, slow
reflex, high blood pressure, and irritated stomach, etc. One
can also suffer reduced learning ability. It was found in
animal studies that young mice and chicks suffer the most
from M.S.G., including damage to the brain and visual
nerves. Based on this evidence, producers of baby foods are
forbidden by law to add M.S.G.. The theory that M.S.G. is a
"brain food" is not based on fact. It actually has the opposite
effect.

The wide use of M.S.G. in China produces some unforseen
effects. Taking a nap after lunch is one. The increasing number
of children with near-sightedness is another. The low work
efficiency and nameless discomforts and headaches are other
effects. I shudder whenever I think about the discomfort brought
on by M.S.G. when I visit China. Ten years ago I visited Beijing,
staying at a guesthouse near the Cancer Institute. I requested
the dining hall to not use M.S.G. in my food. Probably in order to
show extra welcome to a "foreign guest," the cook used extra
doses of M.S.G.. The morning after my first dinner, I came down
with severe symptoms of cold, sore throat and stuffed nose.
Only then was the kitchen staff convinced that I was very sensitive to M.S.G.. From then on they left out the M.S.G. and I did
not have "colds" again.

While visiting Taiwan this time, I learned that the production of M.S.G. produces serious pollution, causing public health
hazards. In the U.S., some Chinese restaurants advertise that
they do not use M.S.G., to attract customers. Many Americans
do not go to Chinese restaurants because of dislike of M.S.G..
Many Chinese restaurant owners are not aware of that, missing
an opportunity to be sucessful.

I hope all who use M.S.G. will change their eating habits after receiving new information. It is also in our interest to encourage merchants to be more concerned of public health than making money. The use of M.S.G. is only a small example of the many bad habits of modern life that need to be changed.

Taipei, February, 1992

Part III

Health of Body, Mind and Spirit

Health of Body, Mind and Spirit

We humans are very complex creatures. Besides the physical body, we have the mental and spiritual aspects. When we speak of health, we cannot speak only of physical factors but should consider the psychological and spiritual factors as well.

The physical factors, are simply food, enviroment, and air. Included also are radiation and enviromental pollution. The psychological factors are emotions, and peacefulness of the mind. The spiritual aspects involve karma of the past and present, and Buddhism. Some diseases cannot be treated with medicine and food. In other cases, although the doctor's diagnosis is correct, and the medication is also correct, the illness does not respond. Often this is related to "karma of the three times." Under this circumstances, unless one uses the methods and theory of Buddhism, it is difficult for the medicine to be effective. If one repents the past and accumulates good deeds, then medicine becomes more effective. Here we will discuss these three general areas.

My Own Learning Process

I think it is best to start with my own experience. Why I am interested in health? What were the steps involved in my moving from physical and psychological to spiritual health? Most people go to visit a doctor when they get sick. Rarely would they look for a way on their own. If the doctor cannot cure him or her, then he would look for an alternative. My health had been poor from the time I was quite young. While in college in Hawaii, I started to think that if I made some changes in my life and diet, my health would improve. I have grown up in a Buddhist family, and have been deeply affected by Buddha's teaching on compassion. I often thought that if we could protect life, wouldn't that be wonderful. I thought of becoming a vegetarian. At that time my parents had the mistaken notion that if one did not eat meat, one would not get enough nutrients, especially for children. They often said: "If you eat no meat, you will not grow up." Under such circumstances, my diet was not ideal. In college I learned that "not eating meat is not enough nutrition" is a wrong concept. I made the decision to become a vegetarian.

Buddha teaches compassion. People usually eat chicken, duck, pork, beef and lamb's meat without thinking of them as life forms. We should not harm them. It was out of this motivation that I initially decided to become a vegetarian. Unexpectedly, my health improved tremendously. The improvement was not only in the physical but also psychological. My physical condition had been weak. In the U.S. I suffered from allergies and hives. The first change after my diet change was that my allergies disappeared. The doctor had warned me that if I did not continue my shots, my allergies would return. Actually in the eighteen years since, the allergy has rarely surfaced. The first result of changing diet was that my physical problems were cured.

The psychological change was more subtle. About six months after the change of diet, I became more detached with the concerns of the outside world. Only recently I came to know the reason. According to the work of Dr. Rudolf Steiner, when one stops eating animal food, the mind reacts to the outside world quite differently. He reported: "If we are taking in animal fat, the body does not need to produce fat. If the food does not contain animal fat, then our body needs to produce fat. Under this condition, the Astral Body which controls emotions becomes activated. This allows the mind and emotions to be free from the outside stimuli, thus becoming more detached and having more inner freedom."

This is the explanation of Dr. Steiner. When your body does not receive animal fat, it needs to produce its own, indirectly stimulating the astral body. The emotions become more independent.

I noticed this change when I was a freshman in college. Students are very concerned about grades. I remember studying very hard in history class but receiving only a B. My reaction was quite detached, compared to before. This happened six months after I had become a vegetarian. This experience got me interested in what Dr. Steiner had talked about: diet change can bring on psychological change. Later, I did research at M.D. Anderson Hospital; initially my interest was focused on diet. It was the same inclination that got me interested in Dr. Ann's work.

I found that this was not the entire solution. After making a diet change, some people do not experience a 100% response. I thought something must be missing.

In 1981, while researching the relation between diet and cancer, I went to China. By coincidence, I came across Chi Gong. One important point in Chi Gong is calming the mind through movements.

Those who practice Chi Gong especially emphasize the balance of emotions. This helped me to understand the relation between sickness and mind. It can be utilized in the treatment of illness, espcially cancer.

In 1984 I participated in Vipassana meditation which started my understanding into the spiritual aspect of healing.

Vipassana meditation was originally taught by Buddha to tame the mind. If we carefully observe, we will find that we cannot control our mind. Even for one minute we cannot ask the mind to do one thing such as watching the breath. We will think of the past, and future events without stopping. This is quite a stress on the body, because every thought produces a reaction in the body. If you have a lot of thoughts, the body reacts and a lot of energy is wasted.

Vipassana meditation is training the mind to focus on the breath, not thinking about the past nor the future. It is conducted usually in 10 days, three days to observe the breath, from 4:30 in the morning to 9:00 in the evening. There is a five minute break after one or two hours. It is a long-term, patient struggle with the mind. The habit pattern of the mind cannot be changed overnight; one has to take it slowly. After three days the mind starts to settle down. At this time, the events of the past will surface, bringing various sensations to the body. Pleasant memories will bring on pleasant sensations. When you think of something or someone you like, you will definitely feel very good. It is quite different from thinking of someone you dislike.

In meditation when you observe the reactions of the mind, you can train to not react. Regardless of whether something is good or bad, it is changing all the time; there is no need to grasp or dislike. By observing with awareness, the layers of stain are removed from the mind. If you continue for seven more days of watching without reacting, after 10 days, you will feel as if a great burden has been lifted from you.

After my first course in Vipassana meditation, I became more aware of the mind-body connection. I also got interested in the chanting of the name of Amitabha Buddha (Buddha of Infinite Light). The Buddha Light Temple in Houston often provide tapes from Taiwan. One in particular is the "Five Intonations of Amitabha's Name." Many of you are familiar with it.

I copied many to give to friends. When I gave these to American friends, they also liked it, probably because of past life connections. It was through some of these tapes that I learned more about spirituality and health. Some sicknesses are due to past life karmas, and others due to spirit possessions. When their physical discomforts are relieved after listening to the tapes, it indicates a possible link to spiritual causes. Here is an example: a friend's father came down with lung cancer. He lived near Washington, D.C.. When I visited the house, I felt a strange sense of heaviness. I started to chant Amitabha and played the tape for one hour before the rooms felt better. The friend told me later: "Our house is built over old cemeteries, Indian and Black slave cemeteries. The area was also a battle ground during the Civil War. Of course there would be many ghosts." Someone with special gifts in the U.S. "saw" the lung cancer connected with spirits.

From all these experiences, it taught me sickness can be brought on by many causes. Sometimes it is only a physical discomfort, sometimes from mental and emotional stress, and others can be traced to spirits or past life karma. If one approaches from all three, then the solution is more likely found. I have introduced my own journey of learning. In the following I will discuss in greater detail how to have a healthy body. If sick how to relieve sickness, following the three areas discussed.

In the Industralized Society, Food Can Be Hazardous to Your Health

First I will discuss food. Food originaly is the most natural thing, not needing much thought. But in modern society, as our eating habits move further away from the natural balance, one needs to spend some time studying it; one cannot simply just eat without thinking. Because of pesticide problems, and food processing, what appears to be better food, is actually food without many nutrients. Every one of you present should understand: Just what are we eating? Whàt effect it has on our body? Only then can we hope to have healthy body.

In 1930 a dentist traveled around the world studying the relation between dietary habits and health. He went to Europe, Switzerland, Asia, the Artic, and Africa. 1930 was a transition time, where the old meets the new. Some societies still maintained the habits of an agricultural society. He found that in those that switched to the industralized society, people's health deteriorated. How did he measure health? Because he was a dentist, he looked into people's mouths and checked on their cavities and dental condition. In the traditional society, he found one cavity per three people. If the diet is changed to so called "modern food," such as canned goods, white rice, white flour and white sugar, on the average each person has nine cavities. From one cavity per three people to nine per person, think of the big difference! The teeth reflect the health condition of the person, because they are part of the whole bone structure. Those with weaker bones will have more cavities. So having cavities is not matter of course, but due to a weakened state of health. Once in Scotland he met two brothers in the same family, who because of differences in diet, also had different number of cavities. The older brother ate the traditional diet and had no cavities. The younger brother was fond of sugary foods and canned goods. He lost many teeth. They came from the same family with the same hereditary factors, so why the difference? The root cause is the difference in diet. This was his discovery.

The change of diet from traditional to modern also produced arthritis, deformations in bone, and increases in tuberculosis. TB was a serious problem in the 1930's. For example those living in the central part of Switzerland and eating a traditional diet, such as coarse bread and goat's milk did not have TB. Those living in the cities had many cases of TB. This dentist found that those who used processed food were commonly affected by cavities, TB, and arthritis.

Fifty years later our diet has changed significantly. During the past few years I have been to India, China, The U.S., Thailand, etc. I have found it difficult to find one truly healthy individual. Every country has different sicknesses. The main cause is the unnaturalness of our modern diet. Why do refined foods increase the number of cavities? The refining procedure remove the minerals. For example, compare brown rice with white rice; what is the difference? Brown rice and rice polishings contain minerals and vitamins, especially vitamin B. After removal of the bran, the resulting white rice contains very little mineral. It is the same with brown sugar and white sugar; the former contains mineral, while the latter does not. One of the common problems these days is high blood cholesterol level. It is the same with Taiwan. Most people think the high level is related to high intake. This is only partially true. The body produces cholesterol as well. When the metabolism is out of balance, then the level will become high. One of the simple remedies is to take molasses, the by-product from white sugar. Molasses is rich in minerals, especially vanadium, which helps the breakup of cholesterol. Sugar cane itself is a healthy food. In our "cleverness," we extract the sweetness and discard the nutritious part.

As a matter of fact, the natural foods such as fruits are sweet and high in nutrition. The sweetness of food is related to the fertility of the soil. Corn from rich soil is sweeter than corn from poor soil. This is based on scientific data. The sweeter the corn, the more nutritious. This is the way nature guides us. We, however, not only remove the minerals in the food processing procedure, but also destroy the health of the soil in agriculture practice.

We all believe in science these days. Science has become the real religion of the modern West. If one is over confident in science, then it becomes a blind faith, trusting machines but not people. Westerners have such a tendency. I remember a study investigating the nutritional value of mother's milk. After much the expense, the result was reported in a paper: Mother's milk is the best for the baby. This is a fact that hardly needs to be researched. But because of over-dependence, science has become blind faith.

Protecting the soil is actually an ancient tradition. Older cultures have their way of looking after the soil. The Chinese farmers treasure the dirt as gold. After thousands of years, the soil is still fertile; it is largely due to the farmers knowing when to let the soil rest, and when to add manure. This is putting back what one takes out. Modern agriculture practices wish to harvest much in a short time. This is due to simple greed, wanting to earn much money. The use of large quantities of chemical fertilizers is for fast growth, for beautiful products and high yields. However, only the major nutrients are replaced, while trace minerals are not. Over time the soil becomes poorer, and poorer. The products are good to look at but poor in taste. When I was young, I remember the taste of mountain apple to be very fragrant. I still remember the taste. Now when I visit Taiwan and eat the same fruit, the taste is no longer there. This is due to lowered levels of trace minerals. So, even is one continues to eat this kind of food, one's health will decline.

I will illustrate with another example: a comparison of tissue mineral contents of Americans compared to Africans found it to be only one fifth. The tissue mineral contents of wild animals of the two continents are similar. Thus this is not due to the difference in soil, but to the practice of eating "modern food." Too much refined food will reduce the body's mineral content.

Heart disease, and hardening of arteries all are related to lack of trace minerals. As I mentioned previously, arthritis and heart diseases are caused by imbalance in food and soil. Let me mention an additional point as to why processed food cannot maintain health. In food processing, whether it is canned or frozen foods, salt is added. Potato chips and roasted almonds, for example, contain salt. Salt is actually a preservative. Traditionally it was used to preserve fish and meat. By consuming processed food, we would naturally take in more salt.

Both sodium and potassium are required by the body, with potassium twice that of sodium. However in modern days our consumption is just the reverse, taking in twice as much sodium as potassium. Our ancestors of 10,000 years ago consumed 16 times more potassium than sodium. From 16 to 0.5, imagine the drastic change! This accounts for many sicknesses. One may think that diabetes results from taking in too much sugar. Although a factor, the main reason is insufficient secretion of insulin. The secretion of insulin can be stimulated by potassium. When we take in too much sodium compared to potassium, that can adversely affect the secretion of insulin, resulting in diabetes. High blood pressure can also be lowered by increased intake of potassium as demonstrated in animal studies.

In normal cells there are specific ratios of potassium and sodium, from 5 to 6. Dividing cells as well as cancer cells contain a lower ratio of potassium to sodium. The ratio of potassium to sodium can actually regulate growth. The long term over-consumption of salt, combined with air and environmental pollution, all contribute to cancer. According to international studies, countries consuming the most salt also have the highest incidences of cancer. The more potassium is consumed, the lower the incidence. Potassium is water soluble. Vegetables and soy beans lose potassium in the canning process and in the making of tofu. What is left is mostly protein.

Plants are the best source for potassium, because they concentrate potassium. Most people do not eat enough vegetables. With affluence people can afford to eat a lot of meat, chicken and fish. Animal products are not good sources of potassium. Even before seasoning, all animal products (meat, eggs, or milk), have a ratio of potassium to sodium of 3 to 5. Slight salting changes the ratio to 0.1 (sodium is ten times that of potassium). Among plant foods, the ratio of potassium to sodium is much higher, usually 200 to 300: banana 200, pumpkin and squashes 200 to 300, watermelon 100, orange above 200, and apple above 200. Fruits and vegetables as well as legumes and grains are the best sources of potassium.

As we mentioned before, food habits in industrialized countries are hazardous to health. Next we will discuss what concerns us most: the question of protein. Most people think that fish and meat are the best sources of protein. Protein is formed by amino acids, eight of which are essential and must be present at the same time to form protein. Two of the essential amino acids are heat-sensitive. In eating cooked meat or fish, much of the protein is destroyed by heat. These two heat-sensitive amino acids are important for memory and energy level. A lack of them can result in tiredness. Plant protein can be eaten raw, such as peanuts, sesame seeds, and sprouts. One needs much less raw protein. Taking protein in the unheated state helps energy and memory. Our requirement for protein is much less than we think. In the past people held the mistaken view that only meat can supply protein. If taken in the uncooked form, we need only one third as much protein. In the U.S. those who are not taking in any animal products still get twice as much protein as needed.

Overconsumption of protein also causes the loss of calcium from the bones. Osteoporosis is unknown among African women who consume much lower levels of protein and calcium than

American women. American women by the age of sixty-five have bone loss of 35%. American female vegetarians have only 18% measurable bone loss at the same age. Calcium is lost in a high protein diet to neutralize the acid residue of protein digestion, regardless of calcium intake. This is one of the negative effect of excess protein.

In summary, the closer the food is to nature and not processed, the better. If you have a small plot of land, grow your own vegetables without chemicals. If the soil is fertile, the result will be nutritious. As an alternative, you can grow sprouts. This is a suggestion for those living in apartments.

THE MIND BODY LINK

Now let us look at the role the mind plays in health. We human beings are complex. Of two individuals eating the same food, one may get sick and not the other. Take the example of Linxian County in Henan province (China). The incidence of esophagus cancer there is the highest in the world. It is generally considered to be due to the eating of pickled vegetables (pickled without salt for about three months until they are covered with mold), and moldy corn bread. They all eat the same kinds of foods but not everyone develops cancer. When questioned, the local residents believe the difficulty in swallowing, an early symptom of the cancer; comes after a particular unhappy incident. This is one example of how emotions can influence the onset of illnesses.

In the discussion on Vipassana meditation I have described how every thought elicits a respone from the body. What kinds of emotions are negative to the body? If one is repressed in whatever way, maybe in one's personality or talents, one will be unhappy. In the East, especially, the parents have great expectations of the children. Some children are forced to study to become doctors, not because of interest but because it is a good profession. On the surface one may be successful but there can be a inner void. In everyday life not being able to express oneself is an important influence on health. It can be seen in the following example.

In the U.S. a pschologist, Lawerence LeShan works on the psychological aspects of cancer. One of his clients was a very successful lawyer. He had a beautiful wife and three children. He appeared to have it all. He was diagnosed with an inoperable brain tumor. He sought out LeShan for help. After some conversation it became clear that his wife was picked by his mother. He became a lawyer under pressure from his father. His real interest was music; he always wanted to be a musician. Even though he appeared to be successful, this was not his life. LeShan suggested to him that since he was about to die from the brain tumor, he might as well live his life. He quit his law practice and started studying music. A few years later he joined a symphony because he had a natural talent in music. His tumor also disappeared. Of course this is only one example.

Another factor that affects the body is not being able to forgive. In life one is likely to be hurt by others. If one cannot forgive, then as soon as one thinks of others one becomes unhappy. If one forgives, then whenever one thinks of others one's heart will not tighten. This is the better course for our mind and body.

Also if our hearts are full of gratitude, we will not be critical and negative towards life and those around us. One of the common mistakes is to not know when we are in grace. We forget what we have and think of only what we do not have. If we are in this state of mind, our body will be under a lot of stress. If we are thankful, then we are happy. The common saying: "Contentment is happiness" is actually a health practice. If we are full of thanks, can forgive and have the courage to express who we are, life will be rich and satisfying for us.

To forgive others is easily said but not easily done. Aside from the ordinary methods to neutralize an emotional wound, one can use color visualization. To love our enemy and those who have harmed us takes special skill. The color sky blue has the energy of unconditional love. If there is an emotional knot in your heart, think of the person who caused the knot and send blue light to the person. Do this everyday for five to ten minutes. After one month or even less your dislike and hatred toward this person will change. Because sky blue light is unconditional love, it can dissolve knots and create a feeling of love. This can be used with those with whom you have difficulties.

Another method of changing one's mind is deep breathing. Mental stress is no more than not being able to let go of this and that, or stop worrying about this and that. Deep breathing can help us let go and relax. When we are angry or worried, our breathing immediately speeds up. Slowing down the breathing has the effect of calming one down. Let us try breathing deeply. Place one hand over the chest and one over the abdomen and breathe naturally. Watch which hand moves as you breathe. Many will find the upper hand is moving, indicating upper chest breathing, a rather shallow breathing. This form of breathing makes one easily tense. If the lower hand moves then one is breathing deeply and is more easily relaxed. In the beginning practice while still in bed. Place a book on the abdomen. When inhaling, push the book up. When exhaling tuck in the abdomen. It is easier to breath deeply while lying down. Repeat 10 cycles initially and extend to 20 or more times. One will find oneself to be more relaxed and detached. Deep breathing is a simple way to change our mental state.

ILLNESS IS RELATED TO KARMA

In the following we will look into health and the "karma of three times." Buddhism contains one the world's most profound bodies of knowledge. Buddhism teaches the chemistry of life, known as dependent-arising. All phenomena are the products of causes and conditions, or karma. If one has studied chemistry, one knows that "things" are composed of different chemical elements. Different chemical reactions in turn produce different products. In the same way Buddhism is the study of chemistry of life. What are the causes of sickness? Generally speaking, if in the past you have caused others harm, such as by killing, the result can be poor health. In Buddhism one is encouraged to follow the five precepts and ten virtues. The basis is simply not to harm others. "Do not kill" is the first among the five precepts. Not stealing, lying, not committing sexual misconduct and not taking in alcohol are all ways not to harm others. Not harming others indirectly avoids bringing harm to oneself. This is the real source of health.

If your sickness comes from not keeping pure morality, the antidote is to take the Eight Vows of Pure Conduct for 24 hours at a time. In the eight vows, besides the ones mentioned in the five precepts, there are the additional ones of not eating after lunch, not sleeping or sitting on large luxurious beds or thrones, and not using makeup, perfume or singing and dancing. Instead of no sexual misconduct, the vow is no sex. This practice can counteract the negativies produced from not observing the vows. Whatever virtues performed in the period of the vows are multiplied numerous times. To accumulate positive energies, one of the best ways is to take the 24 hour Eight Vows of Pure Conduct.

Saving lives is another powerful way to bring health. If our sickness is the result of cutting short of life, extending and saving lives will naturally extend our lives. If one desires health, another spiritual practice is repentance. One such ritual is Confession of Thirty-Five Buddhas. To repent is to dissolve the negative karma. There are actual cases of people recovering from serious sickness after doing these practices. Years ago when I was in India, I often met Westerners with serious illnesses who would come to the East looking for cures. Some had advanced stages of cancer and after meeting with high Lamas they would follow the instruction to save lives, at least the number of lives equal to one's age. If you are fifty, your need to save fifty lives, plus reciting the names of Buddha or mantras. I know of a Canadian woman who had advanced Melanoma. The doctor gave her three months to live. She saved one hundred lives a day for a three month period. She completely recovered from the cancer. This is only one of the many examples. The spiritual practices of purifying negative karma and accumulating positive energies have help many who were given up by their doctors.

One's life comes to an end for three reasons: (1)exhaustion of positive energies or merit; (2)ripening of negative karma; (3) the exhaustion of life energy. If one is forwarned of the impending death, one can do something about it. If it is due to depletion of positive energies, one must actively accumulate positive deeds. Whatever is done out of motivation to help others is a positive deed. If it is the ripening of negative karma, one needs to repent and purify. The following are some Buddhist methods of repentance: Great Compassion Repentance; Confession of Thirty-Five Buddhas; and Nyung-Ne (a two day fasting retreat focused on the Buddha of Compassion). The generation of the great awakening mind, the wish to become enlightened for the sake all beings (known as Bodhicitta) is a powerful method of purification. Bodhicitta arises from great compassion, the wish that no one should ever again experience the sufferings of life and death and all that is in-between. Recognizing that only by becoming liberated and fully enlightened will one have that capacity, one vows to become a Buddha, an enlightened one. If one's life is coming to an end due to the exhaustion of life energy, there are specific meditation practices involving long life Buddhas such as Amitayus, and the White Tara.

If we talk about health, we also need to talk about death. We all must die one day; therefore it is important to know how to have a "healthy" death. The fear of death is stressful. If you are always afraid of death, you cannot enjoy life. On the other hand if you can remove the fear of death, you can fully enjoy life. We are afraid of death because it ends all. We will leave our dear ones and precious possessions. Also there is a natural fear of the unknown. According to the teaching of Buddha, we have died many times. To die is not to become nothingness. Life and death are like changing houses, changing bodies. We have done it many times before. If we have become attached to what we are and have now as "I", then death will mean the end of that. Actually this body is only a temporary residence. If we start to think along these lines, we will view death quite differently.

If you know you will have a good future life, the fear of death will also diminish. At the moment of death, if you are full of love, compassion and kindness, you will have a good rebirth. At that moment it is best to think of the enlightened beings; then you will be welcomed by them. If however you have a grasping mind at the time of death, no peace because of not being able to let go, then you will not have a peaceful death. If we practice not being attached, and accumulate positive deeds, then we will die very easily and peacefully.

Let me illustrate with two examples the importance of mind and spirit on health. When I was preparing to leave Houston for India in 1987, one lung cancer patient came to seek my advice. He had already had a cancer removed from the large intestine. The doctors were going to operate on the lungs in one or two months. I suggested that he become a vegetarian, and find hobbies such as drawing, music, etc. to express himself, and on the spiritual plane to recite mantras. In less than two months his doctors canceled the operation because they could hardly see the cancer in his lung. At the same time he also took up the practice of Chi Gong and Waidangong. He tried meditation but was not suited to it. Instead the practice of Chi Gong helped him release repressed emotions. Another case involved a lung cancer patient in China. Four months before I met him he was diagnosed with lung cancer, his face was blue, and he was ready to be carried to the hospital. Through my relatives he obtained from me some advice given to my uncle when he had lung cancer. He followed it, and by the time I met him, he had no more cancer. If one approaches sickness from the three aspects of body, mind and spirit, one will have very good results.

(From a talk given in Kaoshiung, Taiwan, in June of 1988)

APPENDIX I

THE KEY TO CREATING ONE'S DESTINY

(THE FOUR LESSONS OF LIAO-FAN)

by Liao-Fan Yuan

Translator's note: Yuan was born during the Ming dynasty, in about 1550, in Jiang-Su Province, Wu-Jiang County. He lived 74 years, was a prominent administrator, and published various writings. These lessons were originally written for his son, and have been popular in China for hundreds of years.

The four lessons are:

The Principal of Destiny
The Method of Repentance
The Ways of Accumulating Merit
The Benefits of Humility

Preface to the Translation

China, a vast and populous nation, has for the most part of her long history enjoyed peace and harmony among her people. This is mainly attributed to the spiritual and moral forces that are woven into everyday life. It is too vast a land to be governed by man-made laws, for the emperor had been too far away to rule the people in any direct and effective way. The understanding that "you reap what you sow" or, in the Chinese version, "you harvest squash when you plant the seeds of squash and you harvest beans when you plant the seeds of beans," is deeply ingrained in the Chinese consciousness. This work by Yuan Liao-fan, written originally for his son, is a classic among the Chinese popular spiritual writings. Even nearly five hundred years after it was written, it is still one of the most popular booklets being distributed at all the Buddhist temples and local spiritual centers in Taiwan, the Republic of China. Unfortunately, it is no longer easily available in the People's Republic of China where the expression of her spiritual heritage has been blocked for the last four decades. The value of Liao-fan's Four Lessons is manifold. It provides an insight into the culture of Imperial China and the collective subconscience of the Chinese. Although certain details of the writings were relevant only in the context of Ming dynasty China, nevertheless the lessons can serve as a practical guide to the art of living in the modern world.

The original work was written in classical Chinese, which is poetic and terse. The specific edition of Liao-fan's Four Lessons that I have used for this translation is a Taiwan reprint (1974). In translating into the English, I have followed the original, as well as consulting two modern Chinese translations of the work. The first translation is by Huang Zhi-hai who also provides a detailed explanation of the Ming imperial examination and political system. The second is a far simpler translation by Liu Ri-yi who started a publishing company to print spiritual books for wide distribution. It is a practice in China that spiritual books are printed through donations and distributed free of charge. In a land where eighty percent of the population are peasants, such a practice would insure a free circulation of spiritual teachings. My grandfather was a prominent educator and government official in Hunan, China, and he kept many copies of books such as this one in his home to give to visitors.

This translation has been made possible with the encouragement and support of Dr. David Mumford. It has been a wish of mine for many years to translate Liao-fan's Four Lessons for readers of English, for I have personally benefited from the teachings. This wish is being fulfilled on the eve of my departure to India to embark upon an intense spiritual journey to study with His Holiness The Dalai Lama XIV and other Tibetan spiritual teachers. As a scientist trained in the best of the western tradition (M.I.T. Ph.D. in Chemical Physics), and as a researcher in a major U.S. cancer center for the last ten years, I have become convinced that science alone, as it is practiced today, will not solve humanity's most pressing problems. The problems can be said to be a result of our lack of compassion and sensitivity towards our mother earth, towards the living inhabitants of the earth, and towards one another. Our spiritual development has lagged far behind our scientific and technological achievements, for the awakening of the heart is a natural consequence of spiritual realization. Compassion is the cornerstone of Buddha's teachings, and Jesus taught us all to love our neighbor.

It is my hope that Liao-fan's Four Lessons will be widely read, in the Chinese as well as in English translation, and that the spiritual values will be practiced in a modern context.

Chiu-Nan Lai
Houston, Texas
August, 1987

LIAO-FAN'S FOUR LESSONS OR, THE KEY TO CHANGING ONE'S DESTINY

First Lesson, The Principles of Destiny

I lost my father when I was young. My mother thought that learning medicine would be a good way to support myself and also to help others. In addition, in having a skill on hand one would never have to worry about making a living. Besides, I could become famous through my medical skills, fulfilling an ambition my father had for me. Therefore, I listened to my mother and gave up the dream of becoming a scholar and passing the imperial examinations in order to serve as an official in the government.

One day in my travels I met an elderly, distinguished-looking man at the Compassionate Cloud Temple. He wore a long beard and had the look of a sage. I paid my respects to him and he told me, "You are supposed to be a scholar. You have the destiny to be a government official. Next year you will enter the rank of Erudite (first level scholar). Why aren't you studying?" I told him the reason, and asked his name. The old man said, "My name is K'ung from the province of Yunnan. I have a very sacred text on astrology. I have inherited the knowledge of Shao-tzu (a scholar from the Sung Dynasty who developed a method of predicting the future) and I am told that I should pass it on to you." Therefore, I brought Mr. K'ung to my home and told my mother about him. My mother told me to treat him very well and we tested the old man in his ability to make predictions. He was always very correct whether it was for big events or small everyday events. Therefore I became convinced of what he told me about my destiny, and I started studying to prepare for the examination the following year. I consulted with my cousin, Shen. He recommended a teacher, a Mr. Y Hai-ku, who was teaching at the home of his friend. I became Mr. Y's student.

Mr. K'ung then did some calculations for me. He said, "At the prefectural level you will rank fourteenth; at the regional level you will rank seventy-first; and then at the provincial level you will place ninth." The following year, at the three places, when the examination scores came back my ranking was exactly as Mr. K'ung predicted. Then I asked him to make a prediction for my entire life. Mr. K'ung's calculations showed that I would pass such and such a test in such and such a year, the year I would become a civil servant, and the year I would get a promotion. And, lastly, I would be appointed to magistrate in Sichuan province. After being in that position for three and a half years I would retire, return home to live until the age of fifty-three years, and die on August 14 at the hour of ch'ou. Unfortunately, I would not have a son. I took down the information carefully and set it aside.

Thenceforth, the outcome of every examination turned out to be exactly as predicted. Mr. K'ung also predicted that I would receive a salary of ninety-one tan and five tou (units of weight) of rice from one position before I would be promoted to the next level. When I received seventy-one tou of rice, my superior, Mr. T'u, recommended me for promotion, and so I secretly suspected that Mr. K'ung's prediction was incorrect. But he turned out to be right because the recommendation was rejected by Mr. T'u's superior, Mr. Yang. It was not until several years later that I was finally promoted, and when I calculated the amount of rice I had received there had been exactly ninety-one tan and five tou.

From then on, I believed that whether promotion or wealth, life or death, they have their own time. Everything is predestined. I became quite indifferent about desiring anything. That year after my promotion I was sent to the capital, Yen, for a year. I became interested in meditation and lost interest in studying.

At the end of the year I was to enter the imperial college in the southern capital. When I returned, one day I went to visit Yun Ku-hui, a Zen master at Ch'i-hsia mountain. We sat face to face for three days and three nights without ever falling asleep. Master Yun said, "The reason why ordinary people cannot become sages and saints is because they have too many disturbing thoughts and too many desires. There must be a reason." I answered, "Mr. K'ung has predicted my life, whether it is for promotion or life and death, everything is predestined and so there is no need to think about it, no need to desire anything." Yun then responded, "The average person is controlled by the ch'i of yin and yang, and therefore an average person is under the control of fate. However, for a person who has done extremely great deeds, fate cannot control him. If someone performs extremely evil deeds, fate cannot control him either. For the last twenty years you have been bound by Mr. K'ung's predictions, not being able to change your fate even a bit, and so you are still a mere mortal. Here I was thinking that you may be a sage or an enlightened being." At this Yun started to laugh.

I then asked him, "Is it true that one can change one's fate, that one can escape from one's fate?" Yun said, "Fate is created by ourselves, our form is created by our mind, by our thoughts. Good luck or bad luck is also determined by ourselves. It is said so in all the ancient books of wisdom. In the Buddhist sutras (writings on Buddha's teachings), it is written that if you pray for wealth and fame, for a son or daughter, or for longevity, you will have them. These are not lies because false speech is one of the great sins in the Buddhist teaching, so certainly in a sutra it would be true." I then responded, "Mencius (a Chinese sage who lived from 372-289 B.C.) has mentioned that one should only ask for what is within one's ability, in other words, virtue, kindness, honor are qualities one can work towards. However, when it comes to wealth, fame, position, how can we seek them or ask for them?" Yun responded, "Mencius was correct. You have not understood the true essence. The sixth Zen patriarch, Hui-neng, had said that all the fields of merit are not beyond a small square inch. One seeks from within, in one's own heart, and so one can then be connected with everything. The outside is merely a reflection of the inside. If one seeks into one's own heart into practicing virtuous ways, then one will naturally receive the respect of others and bring prominent position and wealth to ourselves. If one does not know how to look within and check one's own thoughts, but only seeks from without, then even if one plots and schemes one still will not attain one's goal."

Master Yun continued to ask, "What did Mr. K'ung say about your destiny?" So I told him in great detail. Yun then asked, "What do you think you should receive? Imperial appointments? Do you believe you deserve to have a son?" I thought about this question for a long time and then said, "While those who receive imperial appointments all have the look of good fortune, I do not have the look of good fortune, and also I do not accumulate merits to build my fortune. I am very impatient, intolerant, undisciplined, and speak without any restraint. I also have a strong sense of self-importance and arrogance. These all have the look of non-virtue, so how can I receive an imperial appointment? There is an old saying, that life springs from the soil of the earth, and clear water oftentimes has no fish. I have a fetish about cleanliness and so that is the first reason why I do not have a son. The second reason I do not deserve a son is because love is the basis for all life, and harshness is the cause of no life, and I am very irritable and without kindness, too. I am overly concerned about my reputation and cannot forget myself in order to help others in need; I am not compassionate towards others, and these are reasons why I do not deserve to have a son. I also tend to speak a lot which destroys my ching (essence). I love to stay up all night and so I do not know how to take care of myself. These are the reasons I should not have a son."

Yun then said, "According to you, then, there are too many things in life one does not deserve, not only fame and a son. In the world, why there are people who are rich or who have starved to death is because they have created their own fate, and heaven simply rewards that which people have sown. It is the same with bearing children; if one has accumulated enough merit for a hundred lifetimes, then one would have descendants to last a hundred lifetimes. One who accumulates merit for ten generations would then have descendants for ten lifetimes to protect the merit, and those who do not have any descendants are those who have not accumulated enough merit. If one understands the reason for creating destiny, then changing the reasons for not receiving imperial appointments and for not having a son, changing from miserliness to giving, from intolerance to understanding, from arrogance to humility, from laziness to diligence, from cruelty to compassion, from deception to sincerity, then one accumulates as much merit as one can. In loving oneself and not wasting oneself, letting the past be the past and starting a new day, one can start a new life. Once one understands the principles in creating one's destiny, then one can create anything that one wishes. This is what is meant by a second life. If the physical body is governed by the law, then our mind can also communicate with heaven. As it was written in the T'ai-chia book, one can escape the deeds of heaven but one cannot survive one's own evil deeds. Mr. K'ung had calculated that you will not receive imperial appointment, and also that you will not have a son. These are the deeds of heaven, but if you start new ways and start accumulating merit, then you will be able to change your destiny. The "I-Ching" was written to help people to avoid danger and attract good luck. If everything is pre-destined then there would be no point in avoiding danger nor in improving one's luck. In the very first chapter of the book it is written that families who perform good deeds will enjoy good fortune."

From then one, I was awakened and understood the principle of fate, and so I started to repent all my past wrongdoings in front of the enlightened ones. I put down in writing that I wished to pass the imperial examinations to receive an official appointment, and I vowed to do three thousand merits to show my gratitude. Master Yun also taught me how to keep a record of my merits as well as of my mistakes because sometimes the merits will be neutralized by mistakes. He taught me to chant a certain mantra in order to strengthen what I asked. (Note: Mantra Cundi can be found in any Buddhist liturgy book.) Then he told me that I should also learn the art of written mantra, otherwise I would be laughed at by the gods and spirits. The secret to the art of written mantra is to be in complete silence of thoughts from the beginning to the end of the whole process. It is only under some circumstances that the mantra will have its power. He also added that when one prays for something in terms of changing one's fate, it is important to do it in a time of stillness of the mind, then one's wish is easily fulfilled.

Mencius' theory on establishing one's life had stated that a long life and a short life are no different. Superficially the two seem different but without the differentiating mind they are the same. Taken further, if one should live the proper way regardless of good or bad harvests, then one has mastered the fate of wealth and poverty. Or if one lives properly regardless of position in life, then one has mastered the fate of high and low status. To change one's fate for the better, one should first correct all bad habits and bad thought patterns. As a bad thought is formed, remove it from its roots. To be able to control one's thoughts is in itself quite an accomplishment. It is not possible to not have any thoughts but if you repeat the mantra to the point where even when you are not chanting it you are unconsciously repeating it, then its magic will manifest.

My middle name used to mean "sea of learning" but from that day on it was changed to Liao-fan, or "transcending the mundane." It signified my realization that we create our own fate. I no longer wished to fall into the trap of mundane thinking. I changed my whole way of living. I approached life very cautiously and seriously. In the past I had been totally undisciplined, my mind was out of control, but from then on I started to watch what I thought and watched what I said, even when I was in a dark room by myself. Even when people cursed or slandered me, I tolerated it and did not become angry. The year after this, I entered the preliminary imperial examination. Mr. K'ung had said I would come in third; I came in first. Mr. K'ung's predictions started to lose their accuracy, and therefore I passed the imperial examination that autumn which had not been in the original prediction.

When I looked within myself, I thought that I was still not totally comfortable in my new way of being. For example, when I did good deeds I was not thorough, or when I helped people I still had some doubts, or when I performed good deeds but did not always speak properly, or if I watched myself when sober then I would let myself go when drunk. Merits and demerits sometimes canceled each other out. From the time I made the vow it took me ten years to complete the three thousand merits.

After that, I returned to my old home and went to the temple to pay my respects and offer the merits. Then I made my second wish and that was for a son. I also made another vow to perform three thousand merits. In the year "hsin-su" I had a son,

T'ien-ch'i. Whenever I performed a merit, I would record it in a book. Your mother (Yuan's wife), who could not read, would draw a circle on the calendar with the stem of a goose feather when she performed a merit. For example, we gave food to the poor, or helped people in difficulties, or released living things. Sometimes she could accumulate more than ten circles in one day. So within two years' time we had accumulated three thousand merits and again we returned to the temple to pay our respects and offer the merits. Then I asked for another wish which was to pass the next level of imperial examination, the chin-shih level, and also made the vow to perform ten thousand merits. After three years, in 1586, I passed the imperial examination at the chin-shih level and became mayor of Pao-ti prefecture.

From then on I kept my record book of merits and demerits next to my office desk. I also told my staff to keep track of merits, and in the evening I would report to the heavens. My wife saw that I had not accumulated much merit and was concerned. She said that when we were home there were many opportunities to perform merits. Now that we had moved into the official residence there were fewer opportunities. How were we going to accomplish ten thousand merits? One night in my dreams I saw a god who came to me and said, "If you just reduce the tax on the rice fields, that one deed would be worth ten thousand merits." As it turned out, in Pao-ti prefecture, the tax on the rice fields was very high. For each acre the farmer had to pay so much tax that I decided to reduce it by approximately half, but I still had my doubts. How could one deed be worth ten thousand? Just at that time there was a monk travelling from the Five Plateau mountains, and I told him about my dream. He said that as long as one is sincere in performing good deeds, one could count for ten thousand. When I reduced taxes for the whole prefecture, at least ten thousand people would benefit from it. Of course, that one deed would be worth ten thousand. When I heard that, to express my gratitude I donated my month's salary for the monk to take back to the Five Plateau mountains to donate food for ten thousand monks.

Mr. K'ung had calculated that I would die at the age of fifty-three. I had not asked to change this or asked to increase my life, but my fifty-third year came and I survived. Now I am sixty-nine. From then on, I believed that if someone said that luck is deter-mined by the heavens, I would consider the person a mere mortal. If someone said luck is a matter of what we create or become in our heart, then I would consider the person a sage.

In summary, although one does not know one's fate, in times of success one should carry oneself humbly and when things are going our way we should still carry ourselves as if things were going against us. When we are wealthy we should be as if we were poor. Even if we have the love, respect, and support of others we should not become arrogant. If we come from a very prominent family we should not be full of self-importance. When we have a lot of knowledge we should treat others with respect and consult others when necessary. We must always try to help others and yet be very strict with ourselves. We should without hesitation check on ourselves everyday and change any part of ourselves that is not perfect.

Second Lesson,
The Method of Repentance

In the Spring and Autumn Period of Chinese history, during the Chou Dynasty (800-400 B.C.), there were many officials who had the ability to predict one's future just by observing one's words and behavior. As recorded in history, they were also very accurate. Generally one's future whether it will be good or bad begins first in one's heart/mind, and then it is expressed in one's behavior. If one looks kind and sincere and one's behavior is good, one will receive great fortune. However, one who looks very cruel and behaves without consideration for others usually is inviting trouble, so there is no mystery in this. One's heart/mind is connected with heaven. If one is about to invite trouble, one can also see that from their perverse behavior. If one wants to invite good fortune and not trouble, the first thing one has to do is to repent, even before performing good deeds.

There are three ways to repent. The first way is to have a conscience or shamefulness. When we think about our ancestors, the sages of the ancient times, they were also human and yet their teachings have lasted thousands of years. We are only attached to sensual pleasures, fame and wealth, and we have no discipline in our behavior. We commit disgraceful acts behind others' backs, thinking that no one else can see. Gradually one only becomes an animal dressed in human clothing. This behavior is the most shameful.

178

Mencius has said that a sense of conscience or shamefulness is the key to becoming a saintly person. If one does not
know anything about a conscience or shamefulness, then one is
like an animal, and so the first step in repentance is the start of a
conscience and this is what distinguishes humans from animals.

The second way is to have respectfulness. This regards
beings in the heavens and beings in the other realms. We cannot
deceive them. Even if we have made a small mistake, the
heavenly beings and other beings in other realms will know
about it. And if we have made a big mistake, heaven will bring
about a major punishment. Even if one is in a dark room, one's
every thought is known to the heavens. Even if one tries to hide,
one cannot hide one's thoughts, for these thoughts can be com-
municated. As long as one has one breath left, one can repent,
however serious the previous mistakes. There are accounts of
people who have done a whole lifetime of evil, yet at the time of
death, they suddenly became awakened and repented and passed
away in peace. There is a Buddhist saying, "As soon as you put
down the butcher knife, you can become a Buddha." So, regardless of one's mistakes, large or small, the main thing is to be able
to change and repent.

The third way is to have courage and determination. Oftentimes one cannot change one's ways because one does not have
the courage and determination to stop wrong behavior or to
change a mistake. One should regard a small mistake as a bamboo sliver sticking into the skin and one should quickly remove
it. And if it is a big mistake it should be like being bitten by a
poisonous snake and one should cut the finger without any
hesitation. If one can follow the three ways, then repentance will
come as easily as ice melting in the spring.

There are three stages in repentance. The first is changing
one's behavior; the second is altering one's mental understanding from a mental change; and the third is changing from the

level of the heart. Each stage is practiced differently, with different degrees of success. An example of the first one would be if one has killed on a previous day, one vows not to kill on the present day. Or, if one had become very angry on a previous day, one could calmly govern one's inner thoughts on the present day. This is changing one's behavior. However, if one just does this simply from this level it is an oppressive method and it is very hard to truly accomplish a level of repentance.

A more appropriate way to repent is through understanding from the mental level. For example, if one wants to change the habit of killing one thinks about how all living things value life; we should ask ourselves that if we kill them to feed ourselves how can we be at peace? And besides, pain of boiling water and hot oil must penetrate through the bone and marrow. The secret of health is in balancing one's inner life energy and not being dependent on obtaining precious food from the mountains and the oceans. After one eats it is no different from getting nutrients from humble vegetables. Why let one's stomach become a graveyard, reducing one's merit? Furthermore, if one considers that all beings with blood and flesh have consciousness, then the fact that we cannot let them be like children playing close to us is already shameful. How can we further hurt them and cause them to hate us? If we think about all this, then we would be unwilling to kill them for food.

To change one's bad temperament is also the same. One thinks about how everyone is different and how everyone has their strengths and weaknesses; and so we should be tolerant of one other. And when others cannot do things according to our wishes or if they do things against the principles, that is their mistake. It has nothing to do with us, so what is there to be angry about. If things do not come our way, usually it is because we have not accumulated enough merit. So, if we think about this, and even if we are slandered, it should be like fire burning in empty space. It will burn itself out. If we hear ourselves being slandered and try to defend ourselves, it would be like a silkworm making a cocoon, and we would be isolating ourselves. In any case, killing and anger are actions that harm us.

There are other mistakes that we can all change along the same lines. If we understand the reasoning behind the need for change we will not make the same mistakes again. Generally, although one has made many hundreds of mistakes, when you come down to it, it all comes from the heart/mind. If the mind does not generate thoughts that are rooted in selfishness, then we will not make mistakes arising from greed. And if our heart tends toward kindness, then naturally we will not have evil thoughts. This is the most basic way of repentance from the level of the heart. All mistakes come from the mind, from thoughts, and so if we want to thoroughly remove the cause of these mistakes it is just like digging up the root in order to chop down a poisonous tree. So to change at the level of the mind, one should be conscientious in every thought. As soon as we generate a negative thought we should watch and eliminate it. This is the best method. If we cannot do it at this level, then we do it from the level of understanding, and if we cannot do it from that level then we do it from the behavioral level. But the most thorough way is to combine watching one's thoughts with understanding. For those who have made the determination to improve themselves, it is best to have friends and relatives to constantly remind them, or to invite heavenly beings to be a witness and to sincerely repent day and night without rest. After a while we will start to get results, then we feel more at peace and wisdom will begin.

We can expect some of the following signs. Even if we are in a very disturbing environment, we will not get upset. If we see an enemy, instead of getting angry we actually become very happy. When we dream that we are spitting out black things, or dream that the saintly beings have come to promote us, or dream that we are flying in the sky, although many of these occurrences are unusual phenomena they are only indications that we have resolved our past negative mistakes, and that we have made some progress. This is not a time to become complacent.

We average persons make as many mistakes as the many spiny needles on the porcupine. If we quiet our mind down and still cannot see a mistake, it is because our mind is too coarse and we cannot see it. Those people who have accumulated a lot of demerit usually show certain symptoms. The mind is cloudy, forgetful, worrying when there is nothing to worry about, and one appears to be very embarrassed when meeting honest and saintly people, appearing to be unhappy when hearing the truth spoken. Sometimes when people give them things, instead of feeling grateful they would actually become very upset or angry. In their dreams they always have many nightmares. They also complain all the time. These are all the symptoms of someone who has accumulated a lot of demerit; when the symptoms appear, one should proceed to repent.

Third Lesson, The Ways of Accumulating Merit

In the old days, there was a woman named Yen. Before she agreed to give her daughter in marriage to the man who later became Confucius' father, she only asked if the ancestors had accumulated merit and virtue and did not care if they were wealthy. She felt that as long as the ancestors had accumulated merit, their offspring would definitely be outstanding. Confucius (551-479 B.C.) himself had praised Shun (one of the first emperors of China) on his filial piety. For that, Shun will be known for thousands of years and his offspring will be prominent for many, many generations, and these sayings are actually based on truth.

I will give you another example. In Fukien province, there was a prominent person, Yang Jung, who held the position of Imperial Instructor. His ancestors were "boat people" who made their living by helping people cross the river. Whenever there was a storm and flood, the flooding would destroy houses and oftentimes the people and animals and goods floated down the river. Other boats were trying to collect the goods, and only his great-grandfather and grandfather would be interested in helping people and they would not take any of the goods. The villagers thought they were very stupid. After Yang Jung's father was born, the Yang family became very wealthy. One day a Taoist monk came to the Yang family and said, "Your ancestors have accumulated a lot of merit; their offspring will definitely enjoy wealthy and prominence. There is a special place where you can build the ancestors' tomb." So they followed the suggestion and then Yang Jung was born and he passed the imperial examination when he was quite young and received imperial appointments. The emperor had given even his grandfather and great grandfather imperial honors. His descendants are still very prominent.

Another example, Yang Tzu-ch'eng, was from the prefecture of Jin, and was a member of the staff in the prefectural courthouse. He was a very compassionate person. Once the prefectural magistrate was punishing a prisoner, beating him until he was bloody, but still the magistrate was very angry. Yang pleaded with the magistrate to stop beating the prisoner. The magistrate said, "This person has broken the law, how can one not get angry?" And the staff member said, "When people in positions of power have not followed the Tao, then the people do not understand the Tao either, and so they do not understand the law. Thus in a case like this we should be more understanding." The prefectural magistrate then stopped the beating. Yang came from a very poor family, yet he never took any bribes. If the prisoners were short of food, he would always take food from his own home even if it meant going hungry himself. This practice of compassion never ceased. He had two sons — the older son's name was Shou-ch'en, the second son's name was Shou-chih, and they both became very prominent, and held important positions. Even their descendants were prominent for a long time as well.

Another story took place during the cheng-t'ung reign period (1436-1449) of Ming Emperor Ying-tsung. In the province of Fukien there were a lot of bandits, and Mr. Hsieh was appointed to lead imperial armies to pacify them. Because they wanted to make sure that innocent people would not be killed, they managed to get a list of all the bandits who belonged to an organization and secretly gave a white flag to those who did not belong. They were told to place the flag on their door when the imperial armies came into town. The imperial armies were ordered not to kill the innocent. Because of this procedure, tens of thousands of people were saved, and many of Hsieh's descendants as a result became very prominent.

Another example is the Lin family. Among the ancestors there was a mother who was very generous. She would make rice balls to give to the poor. However many pieces people asked for, she would give. There was one Taoist monk who would ask for six or seven each time, and he came every day for three years. The woman always gave to him, and never expressed any displeasure. The Taoist monk realized the sincerity of this woman's kindness and told her, "I have eaten of your rice balls for three years with nothing in return to show my gratitude, but I want you to know that in the back of your house there is a good place where you can build the grave for your ancestors. The number of your descendants who will have imperial appointments will be equivalent to the number of seeds in a pound of sesame seeds." And so in the first generation after the Lin family built the ancestral grave there were nine men who passed the imperial exams, and it was like that for every succeeding generation.

Another famous person was the imperial historian whose surname was Feng. One day his father on the way to school saw a person frozen in the snow. He quickly took his coat off, put it around the frozen man and took him home. That night he had a dream in which he was told, "When you helped that man you helped with a pure heart, and I will send the famous general from the Sung dynasty, Han-ch'i, to become your son." Later the child was born and his nickname was Ch'i.

Another story of a famous person was of Ying who lived in Tai-chou. When he was young he used to study in remote areas. In the nighttime he often heard ghosts and spirits but he was never afraid. One day he heard a ghost speaking, "Because a woman's husband left a long time ago and has not returned, her in-laws think that their son is dead and are forcing her to re-marry. Tomorrow night she is going to commit suicide, and then she will replace me and so I will be able to be reborn." Mr. Ying heard this and immediately sold a parcel of his land for four lien (a weight unit) of silver, and he made up a letter from the woman's husband and sent the silver with it to the home. The mother noticed that the writing was not her son's handwriting, but she then thought, "Perhaps the letter is a fake, but the silver cannot be fraudulent. Why would anyone want to send me the silver? Maybe my son is fine and we should not force our daughter-in-law to remarry." And later the son did come home. Then Mr. Ying heard the ghost say, "Originally I was able to be reborn but now Mr. Ying has interfered with this." Another ghost said, "Why don't you take revenge?" The first ghost said, "No, because of his goodness he is going to become very prominent. How can I hurt him?" Mr. Ying thereafter was even more diligent in accumulating merit. Whenever there was a famine he would take his money and help people, or he would help people in emergencies. And when things did not always come his way, he also looked within himself rather than com-plain on the outside. Even nowadays his descendants are still very prominent.

There was another person, Mr. Hsu, whose father was very wealthy. Whenever there was a famine he would donate a lot of food to others. One day he heard a ghost say, "in truth, the family of Hsu will have a person who will pass the imperial exam." This went on for several days. And sure enough, that year Hsu passed the imperial exam. From then on his father was even more diligent in accumulating merit, whether it was building bridges or taking care of travelers or monks. Then he heard a ghost say, "In truth, the Hsu family is going to have a person who will pass even the higher level imperial exam." And sure enough Hsu later on became the governor of two provinces.

Another person named T'u used to work in the courthouse and he would spend the night in the prison visiting the inmates. If he met anyone who was innocent, then he would write a secret report to the judge so that when they opened the court the judge could question the prisoner and clear their case. So they released ten innocent people, and all the people were grateful to this clerk of the court. Mr. T'u then also sent a memorandum to the Imperial Judge, "In the land within the four seas there are many people, and there are bound to be many more innocent people who are imprisoned. I recommend that every five years you should send a special agent to check into each of the prisons to reduce sentences in order to prevent innocent people from remaining in prison." The Imperial Judge agreed, and T'u was chosen as one of the sentence-reducing agents. One night he dreamed that a god told him, "In your life you were not destined to have a son, but this act of reducing prison sentences for innocent people is in line with the wishes of the heavens, and so the heavenly emperor is going to send you three sons. They will all attain high positions." Soon after that, his wife became pregnant and gave birth one after the other to three sons all of whom later became prominent men.

Another person, Pao-p'ing, was the seventh son of the magistrate of Ch'ih-yang and married into the Yuan family. He was a good friend of my father. He was very knowledgeable and very talented. Once touring around Lake Mao, he came to a village and saw a temple in disrepair with a statue of the Bodhisattva Kuan-yin wet from the rain. He took out all his money, which was ten lien of silver, and gave it to the abbot and said, "This is to go towards repairing the temple." The monk said, "This involves a lot of money. I'm afraid we cannot accomplish what you wish." Then Pao-p'ing took out all his expensive clothing and fabrics and turned them over to the monk. Even though his servant tried to prevent him from doing this, he said, "It does not matter. As long as the statue does not get damaged so what if I do not have any clothing." The monk said, "To give money and clothing is not difficult, but your sincerity is difficult to attain." After the temple was repaired, he came with his father to visit and spent the night in the temple. In his dream the Dharma protector came and thanked him, "Your children will enjoy prominence." Later on his son, Pien, and his grandsons, Ch'eng and Fang, all were appointed to imperial positions.

In Chia-shan prefecture there was a person named Li whose family name was Chih. His father was once a staff member in the prefectural courthouse. There was a prisoner who was sentenced to die but was innocent. The staff member knew about it and attempted to plead his case with his superior. The prisoner, after hearing about it, requested his wife to invite the staff member to her home and offer herself to him in marriage as an expression of gratitude, and also as a way to increase his chances of living. The wife cried as she listened to her husband's request because she really did not want to do it. The next day when the staff member came to visit she offered wine and told him of her husband's wishes. The staff member refused the offer of marriage but continued the effort to clear the case. When the imprisoned man was finally released, both he and his wife came to thank the staff member. They told him that since he had not a son yet, they wanted him to take their daughter as his wife. The staff member agreed and sent gifts to marry her. Their son Li passed the higher level imperial examination when he was barely twenty. Li's son, Kao, and grandson, Lu, and great grandson, Ta-lun, all received imperial appointments.

With regard to accumulating merit, one can go into further detail. There is true goodness, and false goodness; there is the straightforward goodness and the crooked goodness; there is the hidden goodness and the visible goodness; there is the appearance of goodness when there is no goodness; and there is the half goodness and the full goodness; there is the greater goodness and the lesser goodness, difficult goodness and easy goodness. So we need to go further to understand; otherwise if we practice what we think is goodness, but it actually has negative effects, then it is not accomplishing our goal. Sometimes people say, "So and so is a philanthropist yet his descendants are not successful. Yet someone else may perform demerits but his family or descendants are very successful," and start to misinterpret the common saying that the reward of goodness and evil is like the shadow falling after them. This is all nonsense. Often people do not really understand what is true goodness and what is true evil, so one cannot judge by appearance.

For example, just take true goodness and false goodness. Beating and scolding someone, and taking someone's wealth is usually considered evil. Respecting someone, being courteous to someone is usually considered good. These kinds of conduct are not necessarily good or evil, because we need to go further and understand the motivation behind them. It is only then we can understand whether it is true merit or demerit. Popularly speaking, as long as it benefits humankind then hitting or scolding someone is considered merit; if it is for one's own selfishness then respecting others and treating others with courtesy is considered demerit. As for one's behavior in the world, what benefits others is true merit but what benefits oneself is demerit or false goodness. What comes from the inner heart is true goodness; if it is only for show it is a false goodness. If one performs a virtuous act without expecting anything, that is true goodness; if one performs it with a thought of a goal, then it is false goodness.

What about straightforward goodness and crooked goodness? Usually, one considers a cautious and easygoing person to be a good person, but actually the sages think that those who are daring and courageous are truly good. Everyone might consider the person who is careful and weak, without any personality, to be a good person, but the person actually does not have any will and any virtuous spirit. Using this, one can judge others in society as well. Anyway, the judgment of the heavens of what are considered good and evil is the same as the sage's but often-times differs from the average view of society.

Therefore, if one wants to accumulate merit one cannot do it simply by following the way of the world and pleasing other people. It has to come from within where the only thought is to help the world and not to please the world. Truly wanting to help others is straightforward, proper goodness. If one has any thoughts of pleasing the world or playing with the world, then it is false goodness.

Goodness can also be divided into hidden goodness and visible goodness. If one performs a good deed and it is known by others, that is considered a visible goodness. If one performs goodness that is not known by others, then that is hidden good-ness. Visible goodness can only receive the reward of a good reputation, while hidden goodness heaven will reward even more. If someone's reputation is beyond one's true worth, then one will invite great trouble. Fame is not considered a blessing because many people who have reputation oftentimes have it falsely. It does not have true virtue behind it. That is why a lot of families with fame oftentimes have strange mishaps. Therefore the ancient wise men have recommended that it is important to have no more fame than one's true worth. If one has not made any mistakes but is given a bad name, the one who can accept this and not be disturbed by it is a someone with great virtue. Oftentimes the children of such a person will become very successful. Anyway, the difference between visible goodness and hidden goodness is whether it is known or not known.

In performing good deeds, there is also what appears to be goodness that is not actually goodness. For example, in the state of Lu, the law provides that if there are people who are captured by another state, then if people are willing to pay a ransom to bring back the captured, the government usually gives a reward. Confucius' student, Tzu-kung, after he paid the ransom to bring back the captured people, did not want to receive the reward. When Confucius heard this, he scolded him saying, "You are wrong, because what a gentleman does can affect society. It becomes a model for everyone; you cannot do it just for yourself. In the state of Lu there are very few wealthy men; most people are poor. If you start this example of making the receipt of reward money a shameful thing, then who is going to be able to afford to pay the ransom? The tradition of paying ransom to bring the captured back will disappear."

In another example, a student of Confucius, Tzu-lu, saved someone from drowning and was given a cow as a token of gratitude. Tzu-lu received the gift and when Confucius heard this, he said, "Very good. Now people in the state of Lu will be happy to save drowning people, because one is willing to rescue and the other is willing to thank. They created a proper model." And if you use the two examples just mentioned, an average person would view Tzu-kung not receiving the reward money as being very good and Tzu-lu receiving the cow as not being a good thing. Confucius' view is different from the average person. Therefore, when one performs a good deed, one cannot just look at conduct but has to consider other effects. One should not see only the present but also the final outcome. One should not consider only one's own personal gain but how it affects the greater society. If I perform something that appears to be a good deed, yet the final result actually hurts people, then it is something that appears to be goodness but is not. Or, on the other hand, if behavior or conduct is not good but the result benefits others, then the ultimate result is goodness. There are other examples of what appears to be goodness but actually is not, such as improper forgiveness and tolerance; overly praising someone and causing the person to lose his senses; keeping a small promise and causing a greater trouble; spoiling a child and causing later problems; these are all worth contemplating.

In terms of goodness there is also proper and improper. How does one explain that? For example, there was a One-time prime minister, Lu. Who retired and returned to his village. The villagers still treated him with great respect. One day, a villager got drunk and went over scolded him. Mr. Lu was not concerned by it, thinking that it was because the man was drunk so he did not punish him. Next year, this man became even more outrageous in his behavior. Eventually he committed a crime for which he was given the death penalty. This time Mr. Lu was quite remorseful. He said, "At that time, if I had disciplined him then it would have straightened him out and maybe he would not have continued his behavior causing him to do something that incurred the death penalty. I should not have been too lenient with him." This is an example of how a good heart can actually do evil.

I can give you another example of how bad conduct can actually produce good results. Once during a famine the people became violent and began to openly take food from other people. There was a very wealthy man who reported this to the government but the government did not care, so these people became more and more violent, and more open in their behavior. In this situation, the family had to punish those people on their own, and the area had some peace. Everyone knows that goodness is proper and evil is improper. But if one is being good yet causing a situation to worsen, that is improper. Being evil but causing a situation to be good, is proper.

One should also understand what is half good and full good. In the *I-Ching* it is mentioned that if goodness is not full, then one does not become successful. If evil is not full, one does not bring about destruction. It is like throwing things in a container; if one is diligent in accumulating then it will become full, while if one is lazy it will not become full. For example, once there was a woman who went to the temple to offer her prayer and wanted to give something but because she came from a poor family she could only find two cents; the temple's abbot still came out to bless her. Later, this woman became a palace woman and brought much gold. This time the abbot sent only one of his students. Therefore she asked, "Last time when I offered only two cents you came personally to bless me. Today I am offering thousands. Why will you not give me a personal blessing?" The abbot said, "In the past, although you gave little, you were sincere. Unless I personally blessed you it was not enough to reward you. Today although you give much, your heart is not sincere. Therefore I only sent my student." This is an example of thousands in gold as being half goodness, and two cents as being full goodness.

Some time ago, there was an immortal named Chung-li. He was teaching Lu Tsu the art of transforming iron into gold to help the world. Lu asked whether this gold would ever return to its original form, and Chung said that five hundred years later it would return to iron. Lu said, "Won't it cause people trouble five hundred years later? I do not think I want to learn this." Chung said, "To become an immortal one needs to accumulate three thousand merits, and just this speech of yours is worth three thousand merits. Now you can practice becoming an immortal." Therefore true goodness must come from naturalness and sincerity, even such that one does not make a conscious note of it afterwards. And so even if it was a small goodness, it will bear good fruit. If one has a goal for doing good or in giving wants a reward, then even if one performs goodness all life long it is still half goodness. For example, in giving money it can get to the point that there is no thought about it. In giving to the person, it is as though there was no recipient. Therefore, the giver, the receiver, and the money are all outside of one's consciousness. In this kind of giving one cent is enough to neutralize thousands of lifetimes worth of negative karma, and the giving of a pound of rice can bring about infinite merit as well. If one gives and does not forget, or in giving expects return, or in giving material goods feels agony, then even if one gives much gold that is still half-goodness.

Let's discuss the fact that goodness has qualities of greatness and smallness, and difficulty and easiness. In the old days, there was someone named Wei Chung-ta. He was a high official in the palace. Once when his spirit left his body he was taken to the underworld. The king of the underworld took out the record of his good deeds and bad deeds. He noticed that the records of his bad deeds filled up the whole courtyard, yet the record of his good deeds was only a few pages. Then the king of the underworld asked some of his staff to weigh it, the many books of records of his evil deeds were lighter than a few pages of his good deeds. Chung-ta was curious and said, "I am barely over forty. How could I have accumulated so many bad deeds?" The king of the underworld said, "Evil thoughts are recorded as well. One does not necessarily have to carry them out." Then Chung-ta asked, "Why is the record of good deeds heavier than that of the bad deeds?" The king said, "The emperor oftentimes has building projects. When they were about to build a stone bridge in Fukien province you had proposed that it not be carried out because you were concerned about tens of thousands of people undergoing hardship." Chung-ta answered, "I did send the proposal but the emperor did not take my suggestion. How can it bear any weight?" The king said, "Because even though the emperor did not take your suggestion, your intented good deed would have had affected tens of thousands of people. If the proposal had been accepted then the weight of the good deeds would have been even greater."

Therefore, one can see that when one thinks about the world, if it affects tens of thousands of people, and even though the deed may be small the merit can be great. If one is concerned only about one person, and the goodness affects only one person, and even though the act of goodness is great, its total effect is small.

When it comes to difficult and easy kinds of deeds, one uses the same principle as working on oneself. If one starts with the difficult parts then one will not make even small mistakes. Examples of people performing good deeds under difficult conditions are as follows. The Chiang-hsi's Mr. Shu used two years of his salary from teaching to pay for another person's violation fee so to allow that person's family to reunite. In Hunan province, there was a Mr. Chang who used his savings from ten years to help someone return a debt and so saved the person's wife and daughter. Cheng-chiang, had no son when he was old, yet he still did not want to take in a young woman offered by his neighbor as a concubine.

So the above examples of people who gave all they had to benefit others, to understand and consider others, these are all cases where people were doing beyond what a normal person would do or tolerate. This kind of goodness is most special. When one has no money or no power, it is more difficult to perform good deeds and to help others is more difficult, but the merit is the greatest.

If one has money and power, then the opportunity to perform good deeds and accumulate merit is very easy. If, in a situation where it is easy to accumulate merit and to perform good deeds one does not do it, then it one giving up on oneself.

As the common saying goes, "One who is wealthy and does not perform goodness, is like a fat pig."

We have discussed the principles and understanding behind performing good deeds. Now we will talk about helping others through other methods. The first method is to benefit people; the second is to treat people with respect and love; the third is to facilitate the wishes of others to do good; the fourth is to encourage others to perform goodness; the fifth is to help people in emergencies; the sixth is to support public work; the seventh is to give of one's wealth; the eighth is to protect and support the spiritual teachings; the ninth to give respect to elders; the tenth is to protect living beings.

So, as to the first one: what does it mean "to benefit others?" One of our first emperors, Shun, when he was young, would watch people fish in the Shantung province. He noticed that the places where there were a lot of fish, such as in the deep water, were usually monopolized by the younger fishermen. As the weaker older fishermen were left with the rapid streams, he felt very sad. So he decided to join them in fishing, and whenever he met other fishermen who pushed him and took his place, he would let them take his place, would not complain. And if he saw that someone gave him the opportunity to fish, then he would praise him and be grateful. After a while he created an atmosphere of mutual respect in giving. And so, think about the talent of Shun who could easily have used words to teach but he set his own example to change the atmosphere. Therefore, in one's behavior in life, it is important not to use one's own good points to highlight the weak points of others. Do not overtly demonstrate one's own goodness to show up the evil of others, and certainly do not use one's own cleverness to play tricks on others. Always live in humility. If one sees that others have shortcomings, one should be tolerant. If one sees others performing small good deeds then praise them. And so, it will become a silent treatment to those who are evil, but also will not damage other person's reputation, allowing them to change gracefully. Therefore, always thinking about the welfare of the whole and protecting the truth, this is what is meant by benefiting others.

Secondly: what does it mean to have a "respectful and loving heart?" If I were judging from behavior, the difference between a gentleman and a non-gentleman is sometimes very difficult. But if I were seeing it from the aspect of motivation, then it would be easy to tell. Therefore, there is a saying that the difference between a gentleman and a non-gentleman is in their thoughts. There is another saying that the same kind of rice feeds a hundred different kinds of people. Although people are different in closeness, in high and low positions, or in intelligence, they are all people. Therefore one should treat all of them with respect, and respect the ordinary people in the way one respects sages and understand where the average person comes from.

Thirdly: what does it mean to facilitate others to perform good deeds? Generally speaking, in society there are fewer people who perform good deeds than those who do not. Usually people have the habit of defending their own kind and pushing out those who are different. Therefore, a gentleman in this society, unless he has great determination and courage, he has a very hard time making a stance. Oftentimes those who have the motivation for performing good deeds have speech and conduct that are different from the rest of society. They usually are very honest and uncalculating, and do not know how to build themselves up to receive the proper recognition. Therefore, people who lack wisdom oftentimes will criticize these people and so they do not have a chance to perform good deeds. So it is important to support the gentlemen, the ones in a society who have good hearts. It is like treating jade. One does not throw it out like rocks but polishes it to become a jewel. Therefore, when one sees others performing good deeds, one should give them support to help them accomplish their goals.

Fourthly: what does it mean to encourage others to perform good deeds? Everyone has a conscience but the confusion of life and also the attractions of fame and wealth oftentimes cause people to sink. Therefore, in interacting with the average person it is important always to remind others to do good. There is a saying that "to wake people up one moment one uses the mouth. To wake people up for a hundred generations, one writes books.

Fifthly: what is meant by helping people in an emergency? Often in one's life one will be in a situation of failure or misfortune, and so when one encounters others in misfortune, one should treat them as though one is encountering misfortune oneself, and give help without reservation. For example, one can use words to give comfort, or use other methods to help them.

Sixthly: what does it mean to support public work? This is to support work that is for the public good. Building dams and bridges, and helping the poor are examples of public work that one should support.

Seventhly: what is meant by giving of one's wealth? In the teaching of Buddha there are ten thousand ways of developing spiritually, and the first is to give. Giving is also non-attachment. The more evolved ones can be giving inwardly the six senses, outwardly the six worldly phenomena. And everything that one possesses can be given without any question. Of course, the average person cannot accomplish this level and oftentimes sees wealth as more important than life, therefore the first step in becoming unattached is to start giving what is most difficult, and that is money. To help others is to build up one's merit. Inwardly one will start to remove the selfishness, the miserliness, and outwardly one can help others in an emergency which will facilitate the spiritual growth. In the beginning one may feel it is forced, but then it becomes very natural. It will also neutralize one's other shortcomings.

Eighthly: what is meant by supporting the spiritual teachings? The spiritual teachings refer to dharma, the teachings of Buddha. The teachings of Buddha provide a guide to becoming liberated, to becoming free from life and death. In particular when one sees Buddha's temple or sutras one should treat them with respect and protect them.

Ninthly: what is meant by respecting elders? This means respecting parents, elder brothers and sisters, people who are in authority, and especially those who are virtuous and wise. In treating one's parents, one should treat them with kindness and respect. And in working in society, one should not misbehave even if the "emperor is far away." In punishing prisoners, it is important not to overdo it. This all has to do with accumulating merit as the hidden merits.

Tenthly: what is meant by protecting life? The ancient ones have said, "Because one cares about the rats, one saves some rice for the rats, and because one cares about the moth one does not light the lamp." Of course, this is hard for the average person to do, but this is a reminder that we all have innate compassion. That is why Mencius said, "The gentleman should stay far away from the kitchen," (in China most of the butchering of meat takes place in the kitchen) as a way to protect people's innate mercy. He also said that even if one cannot become a complete non-meat eater, one should at least come to the point that if the animal was raised by oneself, one does not eat it; if one has seen the killing of the animal, one does not eat the meat of it; if one has heard it being killed, one does not eat its meat; and if it is killed specifically for us, we do not eat it. These are the four cases where one does not eat the meat, at least to start building compassion and also to expand one's merit and wisdom.

The ancient people boiled the silk cocoons to get silk for clothing, and nowadays when we farm we get rid of insects. As the sources of clothing and food all involve killing, it is important to protect our things, not to waste food and clothing, and so indirectly to protect life. And, sometimes one will accidentally step on things or hurt things with our hands; so one should be very careful. The methods with which one can accumulate merit are many and I cannot describe them all in full detail, but if one could at least start with these ten methods it would be a good beginning.

Fourth Lesson,
The Benefits of Humility

In the I-ching it is said that the heavens will take away from those who are arrogant and help those who are humble. If you look at the way the earth is structured, the water in the higher places always flows to the lower places, and so it is with the spirits and the demigods who will take away from those who are arrogant, and protect those who are humble. It is the same with humans. Those who are arrogant and full of self-importance usually are despised by others and only those who are humble are respected by others. In the I-ching there are sixty-four principles describing three hundred and eighty-four counsels, two-thirds of which are for warning and caution. But in the six principles that belong to the "humble hexagram" they are all for praises. No wonder there is a common saying that humility receives benefit and arrogance invites trouble.

If you look at those scholars who were poor, usually just before they became famous they were very, very humble. A few years back there were ten people from my village who went to the capital for the imperial examinations. Among these there was someone named Ting-ching who was the youngest but also the most humble. I had told other friends that he would pass the imperial examination that year and my friends had said, "How do you know?" I said, "Only those who are humble will receive fortune and in that group he is the one who is humble and very sincere. Only he is respectful of others and does not fight with others. When he is mistreated he is tolerant. When he hears of slander he does not fight back. When one can come to this level of humility, the heavens and the spirits will all protect him; of course, he will pass the examination." When the time came, sure enough he did pass the imperial examination. There were several of the others who did not pass and they changed their previous arrogance and became very humble. They passed the examination later. Before the heavens are going to reward someone, before their fortune comes, the heavens will first awaken their wisdom. Once the wisdom is awakened they will naturally become humble, arrogance will dissipate and fortune will follow.

There was another person from Chiang-yin whose name was Chang. He was very talented, very knowledgeable, and he had quite a reputation. When he participated in the examination he did not pass and he became very angry. He started accusing the examiner of not having any eyeballs. There was a Taoist monk at that time watching on the side who started smiling and then this Mr. Chang directed his anger to this Taoist monk. This monk then said, "It must be that your writing is not good enough." Mr. Chang said, "How do you know? You have not read my writing." The Taoist monk said, "People say that to write well one has to be calm and peaceful, and now I have watched you open your mouth to scold others, and you are definitely not very peaceful and not very calm so how can you write well?" Mr. Chang became quiet and then turned around and asked the Taoist monk for advice. The monk said, "Passing an examination also relates to destiny. If in your destiny you are not supposed to pass, then no matter how much time you spend you will not pass. You first have to change yourself." And Chang asked, "If it is destiny, how can one change?" And the Taoist monk said, "Although destiny originates in the heavens, to build it is dependent upon the person. If one accumulates good merit, then one can attain everything that one asks for." Chang then asked,

"I am a poor man. How can I perform good deeds and accumulate merit?" The Taoist monk said, "The good deeds and the merits are accumulated from the heart. If you always keep your kindness in treating people, then that in itself is a great merit. For example, to be humble does not cost any money. Why don't you turn around and instead of accusing the examiner look within yourself and perhaps you see that you do not have enough humility or that you are not good enough." Mr. Chang all of a sudden was awakened and started to change his ways. Three years later in a dream he came to a large building and picked up a booklet. He was curious and asked someone next to him, "What is this booklet?" The person next to him answered, "Well, it is this year's list of those who have passed the exam." Then Chang asked, "How come there are a lot of blank spaces?" And the person answered, "Every three years in the underworld we do a check and only those who have accumulated merit and have not committed any evil deeds can remain on the list. The spaces where names have been erased are people who originally were supposed to pass the exam but because of recent misconduct their names were removed. In the past three years you have been very cautious, and have worked on yourself very diligently. You may fill in these blank spaces so take care of yourself." And that year Mr. Chang passed the examination and he was the 105th person to pass.

In this way, one can understand the common saying that in one's life one should not do anything that is disgraceful because there is a higher level of consciousness above us that knows it all. So, in one's life, whether one will have luck or misfortune, comes down to one's thoughts: if one can watch one's thoughts and keep them pure (and also watch one's humility), then one will always be protected by the gods and the spirits. If one is arrogant and full of self-importance, using one's power, talent, and wealth to show off or manipulate others, then one does not have a bright future. One will not become anything, and will not even enjoy a little fortune. Therefore, those who are wise and those who understand the Tao will not destroy their own futures or destroy their own fortunes. Only those who are humble can receive the teaching of others, and that is how one can receive wisdom and fortune and benefit a great deal. This is a fundamental understanding of living.

In Buddha's teaching there is a saying that if we want to have wealth and position, we will have wealth and position. If we want to have fame we can have fame. Therefore, when we make an inner commitment, it is like a tree setting down its roots. We should set them down deep, always remembering humility in our dealings with others, always facilitating others, and then naturally we will accomplish what we wish.

Scoring Sheet on Merits and Demerits
As Taught to Liao-Fan by Zen Master Yun Gu

100 Merits
Save one life; save a woman's chastity; prevent the drowning of a child by the parents; help continue the family lineage.

50 Merits
Prevent one abortion; resist temptations (sexual misconduct); provide for one homeless person; bury the remains of a homeless person; prevent one person from becoming homeless; prevent one person from committing a serious crime; clear one person of an injustice; give a speech that benefits many.

30 Merits
Donate cemetery land for a family without land; convert another to the virtuous way; facilitate a marriage; facilitate another in taking the religious vows; take in an orphan; help another accomplish a virtuous act.

10 Merits
Recommend a virtuous persons; remove a source of trouble for another; cure a serious illness with one remedy; speak with virtue; treat servants properly; save the life of an animal that serves man; refrain from using power and wealth for one's own self-interest; publish or edit the teachings of Buddha.

5 Merits
Prevent one litigation; communicate over a lifesaving method; edit a book on lifesaving methods; cure one minor illness with a remedy; urge another to stop the speading of ill words about others; make offering to one saintly person; pray for others; make a vow not to kill; save the life of an animal that does not serve man.

3 Merits

Endure a mistreatment without ill-will; take slander without reaction; accept words that are not to one's liking; urge silkworm growers, fishermen, hunters and butchers to change to another profession; bury an animal that died on its own.

1 Merit

Praise another's merit; hide another's demerit; peacefully resolve an argument; stop another from making a mistake; feed one who is hungry; provide one night's lodging for a homeless person; help another in the cold; offer one medication; give one article on helping others; chant one chapter of sutra (Buddha's teachings); do one hundred prostration for repentance; chant Buddha's name for one thousand times; speak on the truth to ten people; organize projects that help ten people; offer one meal to a monk; provide for one monk; do not turn away a beggar; provide relief for tired animals and people; comfort others when they are worried; for meat eaters to be vegetarians for one day; do not eat meat from the animal one has seen, heard it being killed or killed specifically for oneself; bury a bird that has died on its own; release one life; save a minute life (bugs, etc.); help departed spirits to move on; give money and clothing to people; forgive a debt; return a lost article; do not take improper wealth; help others pay debt; offer land; encourage others to donate to charity; do not take goods stored for others; build grain storage facilities, bridges, roads, clear rivers, dig wells; build and repair temples and statues of enlightened beings; make offerings of incense, lamp oil, tea; give away a coffin; save papers with thousand words (spiritual writings).

100 Demerits
Cause one death; violate a woman's chastity; praise another for drowning his or her child; stop the family lineage.

50 Demerits
Induce one abortion; break up one marriage; abandon another's remains; cause another to be homeless; cause another to commit a serious crime; teach another to do great evil; make a speech that harms many people; steal another's wife or daughter.

30 Demerits
Create slander to dishonor another; reveal private secrets of another; encourage another to sue; break another's religious vow; go against an elder; offend father or older brother; cause the separation of family; in times of famine to save grains without sharing.

10 Demerits
Dishonor a virtuous person; recommend an evil person; flatten another's grave (graves in China are built as mounds); mistreat an orphan or widow; take in an unchaste woman; keep a murder weapon in the household; speak harshly towards parents, teachers and wise people; prepare poison; punish a criminal improperly; destroy writings on the truth; have evil thoughts while reciting the sutras; teach false knowledge; talk non-virtuously; kill an animal that can serve man.

5 Demerits
Sneer and slander spiritual teachings; not clear an injustice when given an opportunity to do so; turn away a sick person seeking help; block a road or bridge; write lewd articles; write a lewd song; speak harshly with others; kill one animal that cannot serve man.

3 Demerits

Get angry over words not to one's liking; scold one who does not deserve it; break up relations through double talk; cheat an ignorant person; destroy another's success; rejoice in another's worry; rejoice in another's loss of wealth and name; wish a a rich person to be poor; blame heaven and others for one's own misfortune; be greedy in making money.

1 Demerit

Cover another's merit; urge another to fight; generate thought to harm another; help another to do evil; not stop another from stealing small items; not comfort another in fright or worry; not care about the hardship of human or animal; steal one small needle or grass; throw away papers with words (refering to spiritual writings); waste food; break a promise; cause another to be drunk; not help another who is hungry or cold; miss one word in reciting sutra; turn away a monk begging for food; turn away a beggar; recite sutras or go to the temples while eating foods with the five pungent spices (garlic, onion, etc., which give one bad breath) or drinking alcohol; eat the meat of an animal that works for man; kill a minute lifeform (bugs, etc.); spill a bird's nest and break the eggs; misuse funds; be in debt; damage temples and statues, etc; use false weights; sell a butcher's knife, fish nets, etc; use one's position to take bribes and other's money; keep lost articles; take goods while safekeeping them for others.

Appendix II

Table of Potassium and Sodium Contents of Common Foods

	potassium mg/lb.	sodium mg/lb.	ratio K/Na
Potassium-Packed Foods			
apricot	1198	4	300
banana	1141	3	380
dates	2939	5	588
orange	662	3	221
peach	797	4	199
raspberries	876	4	219
almonds	3506	18	195
brazil nuts	3243	5	649
filberts	3193	9	355
pecans	2735	trace	>500
corn meal	1125	5	225
rye, whole grain	2118	5.1	423
wheat germ	3751	14	268
pumpkin	1080	3	360
squash, summer	889	4	222
winter	1189	3	396
butternut	1546	3	515
lima, mature	6936	18	385
soybeans	7607	23	331
powder	4150	5	830

Potassium-Poor Foods

biscuit	290	2994	<0.1
bread, white	386	2300	0.2
whole wheat	1238	2390	0.5
roll, Danish	508	1660	0.3
corn, canned	440	1070	0.4
olives, green	132	5770	0.1
peas, canned	435	1070	0.4
bacon	590	3084	0.2
pork, ham	1542	4990	0.3
sausages-cold cuts	1043	5897	0.2
cavier	816	9979	<0.1
lobster	816	953	0.9
tuna, canned	1365	3629	0.4
cheese	372	3175	0.1
cake, plain	358	1361	0.3
candy	9	299	<0.1
crackers, saltines	544	4990	0.1
cookies, assorted	304	1656	0.2
pies, apple	363	1365	0.3

FRUITS:

apple	459	4	115
applesauce	354	9	39
apricot	1198	4	300
dried	4441	118	38
canned	1642	5	328
banana	1141	3	380
blackberries	733	4	183
blueberries	338	4	185
cherries	780	8	98
coconuts	1161	104	11
dried	2667	-	-
cranberries	357	9	40
sauce	136	5	27
currents	1654	13	127
dates	2939	5	588
figs, raw	880	9	98
canned, waterpak	703	9	78
dried	2903	154	189
fruit cocktail	762	23	33
gooseberries	703	5	141
canned	476	5	95
grapefruit	300	2	150
grapes	452	9	50
guavas	1272	18	71
lemon	419	6	70
mangoes	574	21	27
muskmelon	569	27	21
orange	662	3	221
papaya	711	9	79
peach	797	4	199
canned, water	621	9	69

pear	537	8	67
canned, water	399	5	80
pineapple	344	2	172
canned, water	449	5	90
plum, Damson	1234	8	154
prune type	725	4	181
pomegranate	658	8	82
prune, dried	2770	32	87
raisins	3461	122	28
raspberries	876	4	219
frozen	454	5	91
strawberries	714	4	179
frozen, whole	472	5	94
tangerine	423	7	60
watermelon	209	2	105

NUTS AND SEEDS (SHELLED):

almond	3506	18	195
salted	3506	898	4
brazil	3243	5	649
cashew	2105	68	31
filbert	3193	9	355
peanut	3057	23	133
salted	3057	23	2
peanut butter	3039	2753	1.1
pecan	2735	trace	>500
pistachio nut	2204	-	-
sesame	3289	272	12
sunflower seed	4173	136	31
walnut	2087	14	149

GRAINS, BREAD AND PASTA:

barley (light)	726	14	52

biscuit	290	2994	<0.1
bread, French	408	2631	0.2
raisin	1057	1656	0.6
rye	658	2527	0.3
pumpernickel	2059	2581	0.8
white	386	2300	0.2
whole wheat	1238	2390	0.5
buckwheat	2032	-	-
bulgur	1188	-	-
corn meal	1125	5	225
corn flakes	4559	544	8.4
macaroni	894	9	99
muffin, plain	567	2000	0.3
bran	1955	2032	1.0
corn	612	2182	0.3
noodle	617	23	27
oatmeal	1597	9	177
rice, brown	971	41	24
white	417	23	18
puffed	454	9	50
roll, Danish	508	1660	0.3
hard	440	2835	0.2
whole wheat	1325	2558	0.5
rye, whole grain	2118	5.1	423
wheat, red hard	1678	14	120
soft	1706	14	122
all purpose	431	9	48
bran	5085	41	124
germ	3751	14	268

VEGETABLES:

artichoke	780	78	10

asparagus	706	5	141
canned	753	1070	0.7
frozen	1084	9	120
avocado	2055	14	147
beet	1064	190	5.6
canned	758	1070	0.7
green	1448	330	4.4
broccoli	1352	53	26
frozen	1093	77	14
brussels sprouts	1627	58	28
cabbage	951	82	12
red	1094	106	10
savoy	1098	90	12
Chinese cabbage	1113	101	11
spoon	1319	112	12
carrots	1269	175	7.3
cauliflower	1338	59	23
celery	1160	429	2.7
chard, Swiss	2295	613	3.7
chestnut	2059	27	76
dried	3969	54	74
chicory, Witloof	735	28	26
greens	1562	-	-
collard	1819	195	9.3
corn, raw	699	trace	>140
canned	440	1070	0.4
frozen	916	5	183
cucumber	689	26	27
dandelion gr	1801	345	5.2
garlic	2112	76	28
ginger root	1114	25	45
horse radish	1867	26	72
prepared	1315	435	3

kale	1097	218	5
leek	819	12	68
lettuce, head	886	30	30
iceberg	754	39	19
mushrooms	1822	66	28
mustard greens	1197	102	12
okra	971	12	81
frozen	993	9	11
olives, green	132	5770	<0.1
ripe	69	1659	<0.1
Greek style	-	11932	-
onions	648	41	16
dehydrated	6273	399	16
parsnips	2086	46	45
peas, Alaska	1433	9	159
canned	435	1070	0.4
frozen	680	585	1.2
pepper, bell	792	48	17
potatoes	1495	11	136
potato chips	5126	<4500	>1.1
pumpkin	1080	3	360
radish	1314	73	18
seaweed, dulse	36560	9458	3.9
kelp	23918	13640	1.8
spinach	2132	322	6.6
frozen	1606	259	6
squash, summer	889	4	222
winter	1189	3	396
butternut	1546	3	515
sweet potato	893	37	24
taro root	1958	27	72.5
tomato	1107	14	79
canned	984	590	2

paste	4028	172	23
turnip, w/tops	790	144	5
w/o tops	1045	191	5
vegetables, mixed			
frozen	943	268	4
water chestnut	1746	70	25
watercress	1177	217	5
yam	2341	-	-
yeast, dry	9063	236	38
brewer's	8591	549	16

BEANS:

broad	726	6	121
chickpeas	3615	118	31
cowpeas	24554	9	273
lentils	3583	136	26
lima	2948	9	32
canned	1007	1070	0.9
frozen baby lima	1987	667	3.0
mature	6936	18	385
mung	4663	27	173
sprouted	1012	23	44
peas, whole	4559	159	29
split	4060	181	22
pinto	4463	45	99
red	4463	45	99
canned	1198	14	86
snap	970	28	35
canned	431	1070	0.4
frozen	758	5	152
soybeans	7607	23	331
tofu	191	32	6

powder	4150	5	830
white	5425	86	63

MEATS AND POULTRY

bacon(sliced)	590	3084	0.2
Canadian	1778	3578	0.5
beef w/o bone	1610	295	5.5
brains	993	567	1.8
chicken gizzard	1089	295	3.7
heart (beef)	875	390	2.2
lamb	1340	340	3.9
liver, beef	1275	617	2.1
hog	1184	331	3.6
pork	1295	320	4.0
ham	1542	4990	0.3
sausage, cold cuts and luncheon meats			
bologna	1043	5897	0.2
frankfurters	998	4990	0.2
pork, cured	1007	5597	0.2
pork, sausage	635	3357	0.2
turkey pot pie	517	1674	0.3
veal	1450	410	3.5

FISH:

bass (flesh)	1161	308	3.8
carp	1297	227	5.7
catfish	1497	272	5.5
cavier	816	9979	<0.1
clam, soft	1066	163	6.5
hard	1411	930	1.5
cod	1733	318	5.4
crab, canned	4536	499	9.1
haddock	1379	277	5.0

herring (raw)	1905	336	5.7
lobster cooked	816	953	0.9
mussels (meat)	1429	1311	1.1
oysters (meat)	549	331	1.7
scallops	1796	1157	1.6
shrimp (shelled)	689	438	1.6
flesh only	998	635	1.6
tuna, canned	1365	3629	0.4

DAIRY PRODUCTS:

butter	104	4477	<0.1
buttermilk	635	590	1.1
cream half & half	585	209	2.8
cheeses			
Camembert	503	-	-
Cheddar	372	3175	0.1
cottage cream	386	1039	0.4
Parmesan	676	3329	0.2
Swiss	472	3221	0.1
American	363	5153	0.1
eggs	521	493	1.1
ice cream	821	286	2.9
milk cow, whole	654	227	2.9
goat	816	154	5.3
human	231	73	3.2
yoghurt	649	231	2.8

PASTRIES AND SWEETS:

cake, plain	358	1361	0.3
fruit cake, dark	2250	717	3.1
light	1057	875	1.2
candy			
butterscotch	9	299	<0.1

chocolate,sweet	1220	150	8.1
fudge	667	862	0.8
jelly beans	5	54	<0.1
crackers			
saltines	544	4990	0.1
soda	544	4990	0.1
graham	1742	3039	0.6
cookies, assorted	304	1656	0.2
raisins	1234	236	5.2
shortbread	299	272	1.1
chocolate chip	608	1819	0.3
donuts, cake	408	2273	0.2
yeast	363	1061	0.3
sugar, brown	1560	136	11
white	14	5	2.8
pies			
apple	363	1365	0.3
banana custard	921	880	1.0
blueberry	295	1216	0.6
custard	621	1302	0.5
peach	676	1216	0.6
pecan	558	1002	0.6
pumpkin	726	971	0.7
raisin	871	1293	0.7
rhubarb	721	1225	0.6

BABY FOODS:

With the exception of fruits, beets, tomato soup and high protein cereal, all other baby food products contain higher amounts of sodium than potassium.

Note: The above information on potassium and sodium contents of common foods are from a U.S.D.A. Handbook.

INDEX

About the Author:

Chiu-Nan Lai, Ph.D., family origin, Hunan province, China was born in Tainan, Taiwan. She immigrated to the United States with her parents at a young age. After graduating from the University of Hawaii with a Bachelor of Science Degree, she went on to the Massachusetts Institute of Technology to receive a doctorate degree in Chemistry. She did cancer research at the University of Texas, M.D. Anderson Hospital and Tumor Institute for ten years. Some of her published scientific papers dealt with the antimutagenic activities of wheatgrass and cholorophyll, the role of potassium and sodium on reversal of cancer cells, and the relation between bioelectricity and cancer. She lectures frequently around the world on cancer prevention and treatment (U.S., Europe, Southeast Asia, India, Nepal, Taiwan and China). In 1981 under the auspices of the U.S. National Academy of Sciences, she went to Beijing, China to collaborate on a research project with the Cancer Institute for three months to study the relation between selenium and cancer of the esophagus in the Linxian, Henan region. She encountered Chi Gong during that period, and established the Chi Gong Research Foundation upon return to the U.S. to introduce Chi Gong to the West. From 1991 to 1993 she served as the first director of the Land of Medicine Buddha, A Center for Healing and Developing a Good Heart, a center dedicated to the promotion of physical, mental and spiritual health and the cultivation of compassion. She resides in Santa Cruz, California, and Cincinnati, Ohio, and continues to teach at the Land as well as around the world. In response to the many requests from individuals and organizations for information on healing, Lapis Lazuli Light, a global information service network was created in 1993. For further information on the subjects covered in this book, please write to: Lapis Lazuli Light, P.O. Box 1795, Soquel, CA 95073-1795, U.S.A.

ORDER FORM

POSTAL ORDER:

Lapis Lazuli Light
PO Box 42530
Santa Barbara, CA 93140
U.S.A.

Please send me _____ copies of The Pursuit of Life.

    1-4 copies @ 12.95 ea
    5 or more @ 9.00 ea

Sales tax 8.3% for books shipped to California address
Shipping $2.00 for the first book and 75 cents for each additional book
Airmail $3.50 per book.

Name _____

Address _____

City _____ State _____ Zip _____

- -

ORDER FORM

POSTAL ORDER:

Lapis Lazuli Light
P.O. Box 1795
Soquel, CA 95073
U.S.A.

Please send me _____ copies of The Pursuit of Life.

    1-4 copies @ 12.95 ea
    5 or more @ 9.00 ea

Sales tax 8.3% for books shipped to California address
Shipping $2.00 for the first book and 75 cents for each additional book
Airmail $3.50 per book.

Name _____

Address _____

City _____ State _____ Zip _____